adolescent gynecology

edited by **FELIX P. HEALD, M.D.**

Chief, Adolescent Medicine, Children's Hospital of the District of Columbia, and Associate Professor of Pediatrics at the Georgetown University School of Medicine, Washington, D.C.

adolescent gynecology

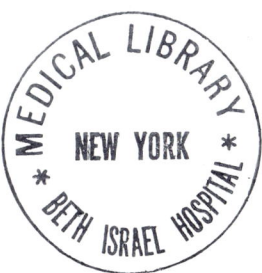

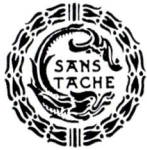

The Williams & Wilkins Company

BALTIMORE / 1966

Copyright ©, 1966

The Williams & Wilkins Company
428 E. Preston Street
Baltimore, Md. 21202   U.S.A.

Made in the United States of America

Library of Congress Catalog Card Number 66–24503

Printed and Composed at
The Waverly Press, Inc.
Mt. Royal & Guilford Avenues
Baltimore, Md.   21202 U.S.A.

Authors Contributing to the Proceedings

Alexander M. Burnett, M.D.
Instructor in Obstetrics and Gynecology, Georgetown University School of Medicine, Washington, D. C.

William J. Dougherty, M.D.
Director, Division of Preventable Disease Control, New Jersey Department of Health, Trenton, New Jersey

Joseph W. Goldzieher, M.D.
Chairman, Department of Endocrinology, Southwest Foundation for Research and Education, San Antonio, Texas

Robert B. Greenblatt, M.D.
Professor and Chairman, Department of Endocrinology, Medical College of Georgia, Eugene Talmadge Memorial Hospital, Augusta, Georgia

Felix P. Heald, M.D.
Chief, Adolescent Medicine, Children's Hospital of the D. C.; and Associate Professor of Pediatrics, Georgetown University School of Medicine, Washington, D. C.

Charles W. Lloyd, M.D.
Senior Scientist; Director, Training Program in the Physiology of Reproduction; Director, Endocrine Clinic, The Worcester Foundation for Experimental Biology, Shrewsbury, Massachusetts

Virendra B. Mahesh, Ph.D., D.Phil.
Associate Research Professor of Endocrinology, Department of Endocrinology, Medical College of Georgia, Eugene Talmadge Memorial Hospital, Augusta, Georgia

Allen E. Marans, M.D.
Research Associate in Child Development, Department of Psychiatry, Children's Hospital of the D. C., Washington, D. C. and Assistant Professor of Pediatrics, George Washington University School of Medicine, Washington, D. C.

Janet W. McArthur, M.D.
Associate Clinical Professor of Medicine, Harvard Medical School, Boston, Massachusetts

Anna L. Southam, M.D.
Associate Professor of Obstetrics & Gynecology, College of Physicians and Surgeons, Columbia University, New York, New York

Somers H. Sturgis, M.D.
Clinical Professor of Gynecology, Harvard University Medical School, Boston, Massachusetts

Sidney L. Werkman, M.D.
Director, Division of Adolescent Psychiatry, Children's Hospital of the D. C., Washington, D. C.

Acknowledgment

The editors have omitted for the sake of brevity the session chairmen's introductory remarks and the general discussion. Drs. John Parks, Andrew Marchetti, Herbert Marbach, William McGanity, and Sprague Gardiner contributed generously from their time and knowledge to the success of this seminar. Dr. Mary Daugela rendered invaluable editorial aid in the preparation of the seminar material for publication.

This seminar was made possible through support by Children's Bureau Grant 214, Department of Health, Education, and Welfare.

Contents

    Contributors.................................... v

    Acknowledgments............................... vii

    Introduction.................................... 1
        Felix P. Heald, M.D. / Somers H. Sturgis, M.D.

1 The Reproductive Endocrinology of Adolescence...... 9
    Janet W. McArthur, M.D.

2 The Biochemistry of Steroids and Hormones.......... 21
    Charles W. Lloyd, M.D.

3 The Identification of Sex Hormones by Chemical and
    Biological Assays............................. 33
    Joseph W. Goldzieher, M.D.

4 Metropathia Hemorrhagica and Nonpsychogenic
    Amenorrhea................................. 45
    Annd L. Southam, M.D.

5 The Management of Congenital Defects............. 58
    Somers H. Sturgis, M.D.

6 Ovarian Tumors During Adolescence................ 69
    Felix P. Heald, M.D.

7 Hirsutism....................................... 77
    *Virendra B. Mahesh, Ph.D., D.Phil. and Robert
    B. Greenblatt, M.D.*

8 Vaginitis....................................... 104
    Alexander M. Burnett, M.D

CONTENTS

9 Public Health Aspects of Venereal Disease............ 109
   William J. Dougherty, M.D.

10 The Psychological Impact of Pregnancy on the Adolescent Girl
   Allen E. Marans, M.D.

11 Sex Education in Adolescence........................ 130
   Sidney L. Werkman, M.D.

Index.. 149

Introduction

Felix P. Heald, M.D.

This meeting inaugurates the first of a series of projected seminars over the next few years which will have as their primary function discussion of many different aspects of the adolescent. The adolescent has always been a very attractive subject for discussion and investigation. Interest in the adolescent began to shift from primarily psychological focus to a medical-psychological orientation with the establishment of a medical unit for adolescents at the Children's Hospital in Boston in 1951. With Dr. J. Roswell Gallagher as its head, it stimulated wide interest throughout this country. To numerous groups interested in the medical aspects of care of adolescents, it seemed quite logical to establish a forum to which they could come and freely discuss the important medical, psychological, and social aspects of the teenager.

To set the stage for the beginning of this seminar properly, adolescence should be defined. The Universal Oxford Dictionary defines adolescence as follows: "The process or condition of growing up; the growing age, youth period between childhood and maturity, extending from 14 to 25 in males and from 12 to 21 in females." From an administrative standpoint, the adolescent unit at the Children's Hospital of the District of Columbia is limited to those youngsters between the ages of 12 and 21. These age limits are similar in the unit in Boston. In general the lower age limit for most adolescent units that I am aware of in this country is 12 years with the upper age limit varying from 17 to 21. As you noticed, I have used the term, administrative, since a closer look at the biology of adolescence clearly indicates that the lower age limit for adolescence certainly is not age 12. The endocrine and body compositional changes that signify adolescence appear to begin between the 8th and 10th year in both boys and girls with changes indicating the beginning of adolescence most clearly defined in the girl certainly by the age of 10. It would seem then that a biological definition of adolescence would certainly begin with age 10 and cease with the termination of growth, generally girls by the 17th year and boys by the 19th year. It appears reasonable to define the period of adolescence, from a biological standpoint, as being between the ages of 10 and 19 years. This upper age limit functions well in our own adolescent clinic since most youngsters are willing to come to the adolescent clinic through high school. Once they have finished high school, unless they have been carried in our division for a long time and have a special attachment to our unit, few adolescents are seen in our division.

During the next several days, we may be hearing about prevalence rates for disorders of the adolescent girl. It may come as a surprise to some of you to know the magnitude of the adolescent population in the United States. In 1962 there were 32½ million youngsters between the ages of 10 and 19. In regard to gynecological disorders, approximately one-half of the 32½ million will be girls and a goodly number of these will have already had the menarche. For the first time the reproductive system of the female then becomes the object of scrutiny to the emerging young lady, her parents, and her physician. The problem that has plagued physicians is to distinguish between normality of erratic early menstrual function and those abnormalities of menstruation which require identification and treatment. The tendency has been to assume that erratic menstrual function early in adolescence reflects immaturity of the reproductive system and, as Dr. McArthur has stressed, that a physician must wait patiently until sufficient menstrual experience has accumulated to allow a more regular and cyclical menstruation. The recent work of Dr. Southam has caused the physician to pause and reflect on the possibility that erratic menstruation early in adolescence may be the indicator of severe problems in ovarian function and later in fertility. The physician must be very wary of resorting to the adage that is so commonly applied to disorders of children and adolescents—"they will grow out of it." When a clearer natural

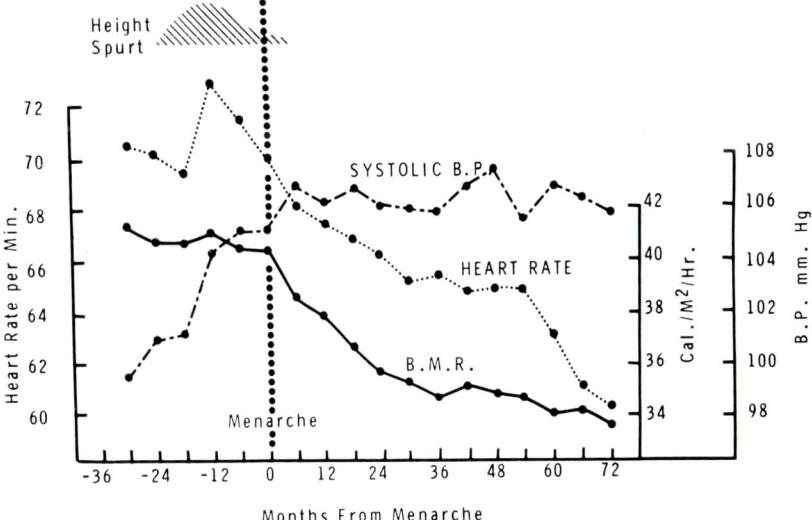

FIG. I. The general relationship between selected physiological parameters to sexual maturation (in this case, menarche) during the adolescent growth spurt.

history and characterization of specific gynecological disorders are available to us, their identification in the adolescent girl and decisions related to treatment will become a more integral part of adolescent medicine.

Finally, it would be remiss of me not to stress the importance of menarche as a biological marker in developmental and metabolic research during adolescence. Many of the sex differences in body composition, physiology, and metabolism that develop in human biology make their appearance during the adolescent growth spurt. Early emphasis, particularly by Dr. William Greulich, was placed on relating physiological data to the biological or maturational status of the subject. The use of biological maturation rather than chronological age as an index of development results in a clearer definition of the physiological and metabolic changes in adolescence. There are numerous examples in the literature which indicate that introducing biological maturation into the experimental design of a study results in data which make better physiological sense. Figure I plots some very simple physiological parameters such as heart rate, oxygen consumption, and blood pressure measured longitudinally in an adolescent girl.[1]

For example, oxygen consumption declines through the period of growth and adult life. The only time this decline is temporarily interrupted is during adolescence. The fall in pulse rate and the rise in systolic blood pressure both are clearly related to the onset of menarche. These are relatively simple examples of an important phenomenon, which is the relationship of menarche to physiological and metabolic parameters. These are some reflections concerning adolescence and, in particular, the adolescent girl; and since we are all anxious to go on with the seminar, Dr. Somers H. Sturgis, the Co-Chairman, has some remarks before the beginning of our seminar.

REFERENCE

1. Tanner, J. M.: *Growth at Adolescence,* Ed. 1, p. 156, Fig. 32. Blackwell Scientific Publications, Publisher, Oxford, England, 1962.

Introduction

Somers H. Sturgis, M.D.

I suppose that in the definitions of adolescence that Dr. Heald gave us this morning there could be as many variations as there are registrants in this course. Certainly, as he pointed out, neither biologically nor chronologically have we any way to set a definite limit on adolescence to which we would all agree. There must be other ways of doing it. The facetious among us might agree that this is the time at which we are trying to keep our young girls off their backs. Others have more psychological ideas of defining adolescence, and to this we are going to apply ourselves this afternoon. The psychological definition might be the time in which a boy or girl is trying to establish his own personality structure and mature identity.

The adolescent girl whom we're going to be considering these three days is a lost soul medically and has been so for many years. Pediatricians generally don't have the background or experience to follow her through the middle teens to the late teens with the knowledge of her hormone, endocrine, and psychological behavior patterns. Often enough in the past she has been sent to the best obstetrician-gynecologist in the neighborhood and he, being very successful and having little time to give to her problems, admits her for a D and C the next day; this is his only answer to a problem of bleeding. It seems surprising that adolescent medicine has taken so long to gell into a speciality. Geriatrics has been with us for some years. It certainly is appropriate now to see a sudden surge of interest in adolescent medicine *per se* as a limited discipline in medicine that has its own criteria for definition and treatment.

The pediatrician has had a bible for long years. All he needs to do when any problem comes up is to open Dr. Spock to page 455 and find the answer. We don't have a Dr. Spock for adolescent medicine; I'm not sure whether Dr. Gallagher or Dr. Heald is going to be the author of some such, but we need it. We are still new in this discipline. We still have a lot to learn. Yet the adolescent presents a tremendous challenge to both parents and physicians. I speak as a parent of three daughters in saying that as a guidance specialist to my daughters, I'm no good at all. And perhaps other parents here will agree with me. My children don't listen to me. I don't know what to do with their problems. And it seems to me that one of the parameters of adolescent medicine may well be the willingness to accept the fact that those of you who are going to dedicate yourselves to this group also have a tremendous opportunity for parental guidance.

The pattern, after all, is set by the adolescent both medically and socially and is going to be pretty well fixed by the late teens when he or she goes off to college or gets married and gets a job—gets out from under parental guidance. By this time the parent has little or nothing to do with the direction of his daughter's life.

We all recognize that adolescents give us the greatest opportunity to mold, direct, or influence the patterns of behavior that may become fixed and irreversible later on. Yet, as we got an inkling this morning, there are numbers of problems that we simply don't know the answers to. These are matters for discussion and research.

How important, for instance, is heredity in the problem of obesity or hirsutism, dysmenorrhea, or immaturity? How important is it to correct anovulation in the youngster? What about premenstrual tension? Are we at liberty to curb the too rapid growth of the 16-year-old girl who now is already 5 feet 10 inches tall and anticipating a lifetime of overlooking her male companions? Does it do any harm to fuse the epiphyses with steroids which do so many metabolic things to the youngster? Can we permanently benefit a girl by doing a presacral section for dysmenorrhea? Are we at liberty to suppress ovulation for long periods of time in patients 15 or 16 years old? These are samples of the questions that all of us need to have answered, and certainly those of you in adolescent medicine are going to have a chance to answer them.

In the office of a gynecologist are seen the end results of adolescent patterns that he cannot help feeling might have been reversed if they had been approached early enough. Take, for instance, the polycystic ovary syndrome mentioned this morning. There is no doubt at all in any of our minds that somewhere along the line the development of a polycystic ovary must have started. And there is certainly a good deal of feeling that if we could diagnose this at an early age then we ought to be able to do something about it, to reverse the situation before this girl comes in in her twenties as an infertility patient and has to have a wedge resection.

There must be some way to determine the onset of endocrine imbalances and situations such as the polycystic ovary syndrome in adolescence.

We also have to deal with infertility. In a couple's twenties or maybe early thirties, the usual conservative idea is that they should have 2 years of sexual exposure before the fancy studies for infertility. More liberally we may wait for only 1 year of exposure, but the problems that we see in infertility include frigidity, dyspareunia, and all sorts of states of marital unhappiness. Those problems were inherent in the adolescent, probably long before she ever got married. For this reason, I have to advance the plea for using the premarital examination to try to do some prophylactic work to eliminate the unhappiness and sordid figures of induced abortion and illegitimate children of unmarried mothers and all the rest that is plaguing America today.

I suppose that one has to agree that churches, parents, and social groups have not done a very good job on indoctrination in the responsibilities of mature sex. And I think the medical profession must take a more active part in trying to reverse the statistics that are really pretty horrible in this country.

The premarital examination is one of the God-given opportunities for us to do something about this. In general, the local doctor or general practitioner does a blood test and that's all. Unfortunately, too many obstetricians and gynecologists don't take this opportunity to try to size up a youngster when she comes in for a blood test. As adolescent medicine recruits more and more physicians, premarital counseling will become part of their specialty. You are going to see teen-age patients coming in for premarital exams and this is your opportunity to accept this challenge. You can so easily do this by the instinctive evaluation of the young girl, when she comes in for a blood test. Give her a chance to talk and show how much she does or doesn't know, or is or isn't prepared for the responsibilities of married life in regard to sexual function. Of course, it is not easy for any of us to give the time to do anything about the case of a totally irresponsible or unsophisticated youngster who comes in a month before marriage. But still it will give us the opportunity to make our own mental note to evaluate the need of this youngster for help, so that we can get hold of her, have her come back, and take some steps about it later on. So, this, again, is one of the aspects of adolescent medicine that we must include in addition to the other challenges of this particular discipline.

1

The Reproductive Endocrinology of Adolescence*

Janet W. McArthur, M.D.

Adolescence, a dynamic period which culminates in the attainment of full reproductive competence, is one of the most meagerly documented epochs from the physiological point of view. The pseudoprecocious neonate with its temporary surfeit of maternal estrogens and the postmenopausal woman with her high titer of gonadotropic hormones have lent themselves readily to endocrine definition. No so the adolescent, in whom documentation is an arduous undertaking, requiring not only the use of ultrasensitive techniques but their application in longitudinal studies conducted over an extended period of time.

The overt physical response to the increasing hormone production of the premenarcheal years has been described elsewhere.[10, 11, 18] What will be undertaken here is a description of the hormonal changes which immediately precede and follow the menarche, and of the subtle but real impact of these changes upon reproductive function.

In girls between the ages of 1 and 9 years, follicles at all stages of development and atresia are constantly present in the ovaries.

---

* From the Department of Medicine, Harvard Medical School, Boston, Mass. This study was supported in part by the Barbara C. Wilcox Fund, the Sprague Fund, and Research Grant AM 04378-05 from the United States Public Health Service.

However, the Graafian follicles tend to be small, the largest rarely attaining a diameter greater than 2 mm. Alkaline phosphatase activity, which is scarcely demonstrable in the theca cells of the adult ovary prior to the appearance of an antrum, is seldom evident in the theca interna of children's ovaries. However, after the age of 9, there is a noticeable increase in the size of the follicles, and alkaline phosphatase activity appears in the luteinized theca interna cells in concentrations approaching those of the adult.[16] In rats, development of the follicles to the antrum stage can occur without the mediation of pituitary hormones, being demonstrable in the hypophysectomized animals; development beyond the antrum stage, on the other hand, cannot proceed without gonadotropic stimulation.

From these anatomical considerations, one might anticipate that gonadotropic and estrogenic activity, if present at all, would be demonstrable only with difficulty in girls up to the age of 9 and would thereafter exhibit a progressive increase. The recent study of Fitschen and Clayton,[6] utilizing human chorionic gonadotropin (HCG)-augmented mouse uterine weight as the response parameter, has validated this prediction with respect to gonadotropins. Their method, although not specific for either the follicle-stimulating hormone (FSH) or the luteinizing hormone (LH), is sufficiently sensitive to permit the intermittent detection of gonadotropic activity in 75 per cent of girls in the 0 to 6 year age group (Fig. 1.1). The levels found in girls are generally lower than those found in boys of the same age. Higher levels begin to be detected in girls 9 to 10 years of age, and in the pooled urine of postmenarcheal females the level is distinctly higher than in premenarcheal girls, there being no overlapping of the fiducial limits.

Data concerning the excretion of FSH and LH in puberty are few. Utilizing a technique thought to measure FSH specifically, Brown[2] found surprisingly high levels in girls of the 10 to 11 year age group. The concentration of FSH per liter fell with increasing age. Unfortunately, it is not clear whether this observation is attributable to increasing urine volumes in older children or to a higher level of FSH in the circulation of younger children.

Employing the ovarian ascorbic acid depletion method, thought to be relatively specific for LH, Fitschen and Clayton found

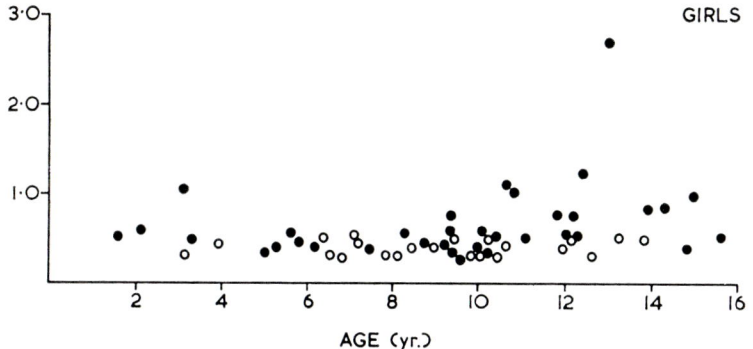

Fig. 1.1. The urinary excretion of gonadotropic activity in girls. Dots correspond to measurable levels, expressed in milligrams I.R.P. per 24 hours; open circles indicate failure to detect gonadotropic activity and an excretion level below the value indicated. From Fitschen and Clayton.[6]

measurable quantities of LH in the pooled urine of girls of all age groups, the amount increasing with age. Only sluggish oscillations in the level of LH were observed during the menstrual cycle of a 15-year-old girl studied with the aid of the prostatic weight method by McArthur and associates (Fig. 1.2); the burst of LH excretion which occurs characteristically during midcycle in adult women was absent.

Biological assays of urinary estrogens in childhood and adolescence have revealed barely detectable amounts (presumably of adrenal origin) below the age of 7, a slight increase in both sexes between the ages of 7 and 8, and a marked increase in girls between the ages of 11 and 12 (Fig. 1.3). The advent of cyclicity in estrogen excretion presages the occurrence of the menarche.

Chemical assays of the three "classic" estrogens have been performed on the urine of 9- to 11-year-old children of both sexes (Table 1.1). They reveal a slightly higher level of total estrogens and, in particular, of estriol, in girls than in boys. Excretion levels of estrone, estradiol, and estriol were found to be considerably lower during the ovulatory menstrual cycle of a 17-year-old girl than during that of a 32-year-old woman (Fig. 1.4). Data which would establish whether secretion of the classic estrogens is regularly higher in adult women than in adolescent girls have not yet been obtained; a description of the qualitative changes in sex

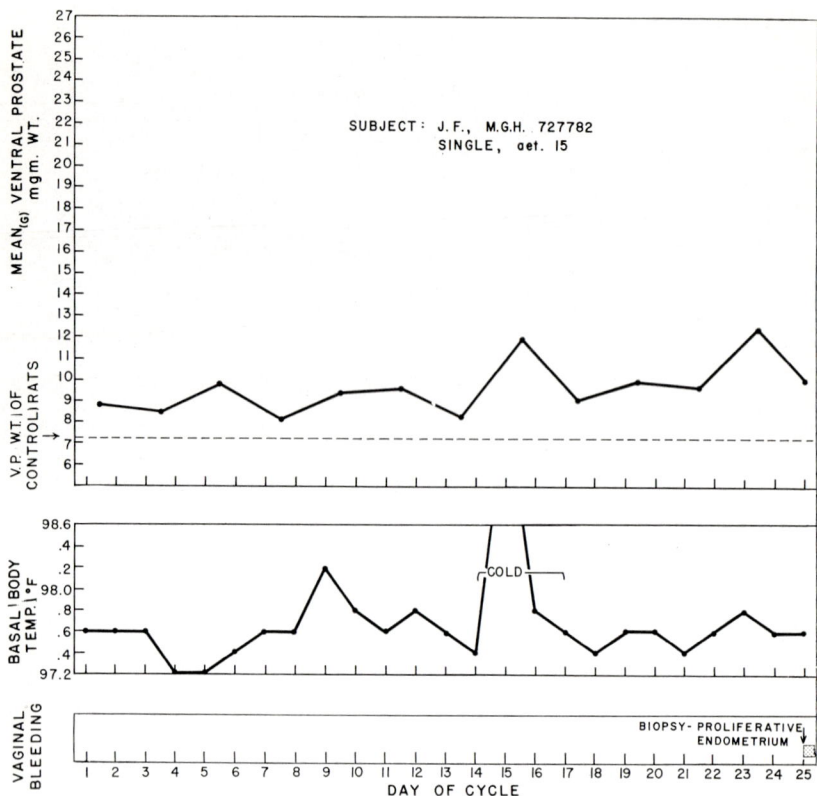

Fig. 1.2. The mean ventral prostatic weight in hypophysectomized immature male rats treated with the equivalent of 6 hours of urine of a 15-year-old girl during an anovulatory cycle. Each point represents the mean response of three animals. Adapted from McArthur and associates.[12]

steroid secretion during maturation is, in addition, unavailable. It is likely, however, that the changes in sex steroid secretion which occur during adolescence are not solely quantitative in character.

Once a bolt of LH is released in midcycle and effects the ovulation of a suitably primed follicle, increased quantities of pregnandiol become suddenly detectable in the urine. However, the duration of the luteal phase tends to be foreshortened relative to that of the adult organism. With advancing age, ovulation occurs with greater frequency (Table 1.2) and the luteal phase length-

REPRODUCTIVE ENDOCRINOLOGY OF ADOLESCENCE

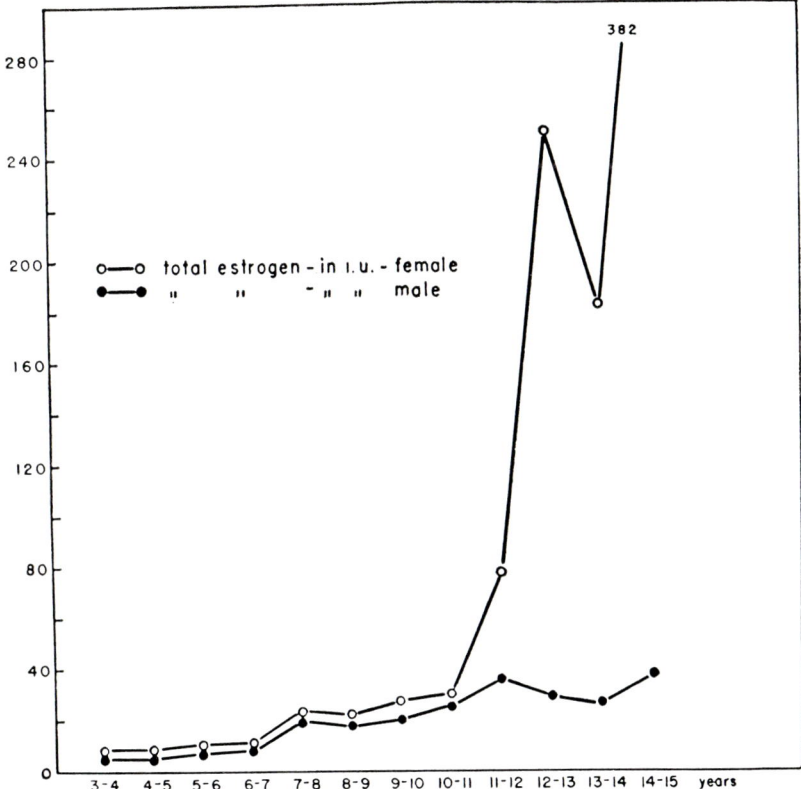

Fig. 1.3. The urinary excretion of total estrogens in international units by boys and girls of different ages. From Nathanson and associates.[14]

TABLE 1.1

*The Urinary Excretion of Estrogens by Immature Boys and Girls**

	No.	Age	Estrone	Estradiol	Estriol
		yrs.	μg./ 24 hrs.		
Girls	12	9–11	0.9	0.5	1.0
Boys	7	10–12	0.6	1.1	0.2

* The urinary excretion of estrone, estradiol, and estriol as measured by the Brown method in 19 girls and boys between the ages of 9 and 12 years. These values lie at the lower limit of sensitivity, especially the estriol levels in boys. From Persson.[15]

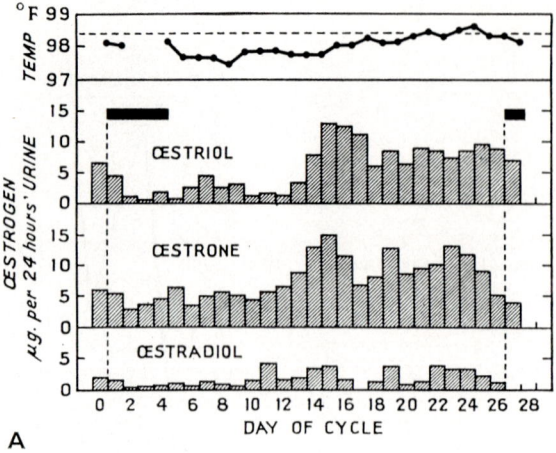

Fig. 1.4. Charts showing the day-to-day changes in basal body temperature and in the urinary excretion of estriol, estrone and estradiol throughout: A, a 26-day menstrual cycle in a 17-year-old subject; and B, a 28-day cycle in a 32-year-old para II subject. From Brown.[1]

ens, as adjudged by the configuration of the basal body temperature curve (Fig. 1.5). Direct measurements of urinary pregnandiol show that the luteal level increases with each succeeding decade (Fig. 1.6). According to the *in vitro* studies of Savard and associates,[17] LH is the only luteotropic agent operative in the nonpregnant human female. It seems likely, therefore, that the luteal insufficiency of adolescence, both as regards duration and intensity, is ascribable to deficient LH secretion.

The reproductive consequences of LH deficiency are more readily assessed in experimental animals than in human beings. In 100 adolescent female mice run with mature males at the first estrus, only 24 conceived, whereas 80 to 90 per cent conceived when mated at the age of 3 to 6 months.[13] Among primates, the chimpanzee lends itself particularly well to such studies inasmuch as its 38-day menstrual cycle is divisible into four externally recognizable phases. These are as follows: menstruation, 3 days; a preswelling phase or interval period of ovarian follicular inactivity, 7 days; a phase of swelling of the sexual skin corresponding to the follicular phase, 18 days; and a postswelling phase corresponding to the luteal phase, 10 days. As maturation proceeds, the preswelling and swelling phases and menstruation become

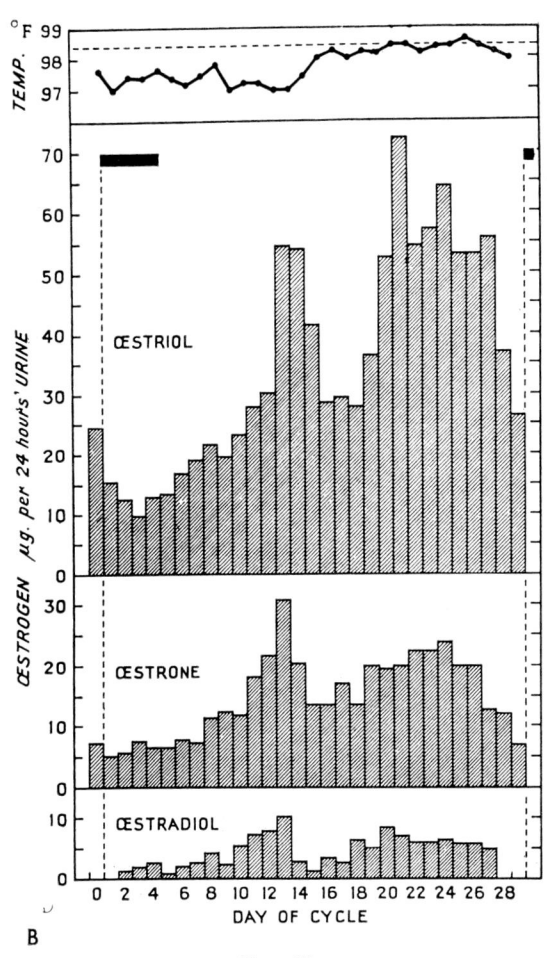

Fig. 4B

TABLE 1.2

The Incidence of Anovulatory Cycles in Women of Different Ages

Age	No. of Subjects	No. of Cycles	Anovulatory Cycles	
yrs.			no.	%
17–19	59	81	25	30.8
20–24	33	112	11	9.8
25–29	21	45	2	4.4
30–34	11	23	0	0
35–39	13	33	4	12.1
40–50	11	33	5	15.1

* The incidence of anovulatory cycles, as adjudged by the basal body temperature pattern derived from 327 cycles of 148 subjects ranging in age from 17 to 50 years and subdivided into groups as shown. From Collett and associates.[3]

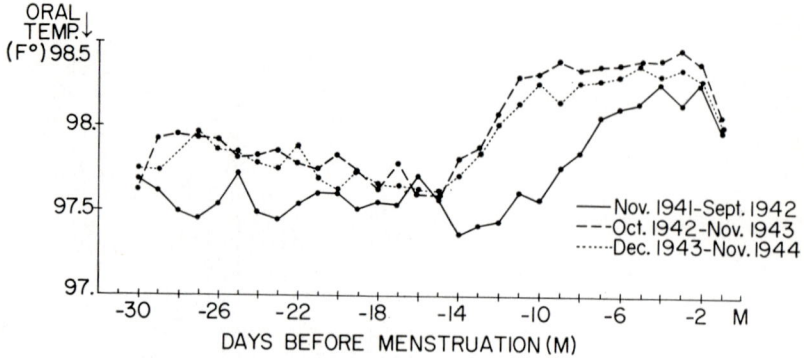

Fig. 1.5. Chart showing the mean basal body temperature for each of 3 successive years in a normal girl who recorded her basal body temperature daily, beginning after the second menstrual period at the age of 12 years and 6 months. The mean temperatures have been computed after grouping each month's figures according to the number of days prior to the menstrual period. The waking temperatures during the 1st year differ from those of the 2nd and 3rd years, which are similar. During the 1st year, there is no sharp break in the temperature curve at the approximate time of ovulation, whereas in the 2nd and 3rd years there is a sharp break on Day −10. The 1st year's records show a gradual rise beginning at the estimated time of ovulation, and this eventually approaches the level of the 2nd and 3rd years. However, instead of the rise taking place over a period of 48 hours, as is usual in the adolescent, it requires a period of 7 or 8 days. The curve is not the result of averaging typical ovulatory and anovulatory curves but is typical in itself. It is characterized by a gradual rise in temperature over a period of a week, starting at the estimated time of ovulation. From Cooperman.[4]

shorter, and the postswelling phase becomes longer. The results of timed matings are summarized in Table 1.3. It will be noted that with increasing age the proportion of fertile matings increases and early abortions become more infrequent. Although ovulation evidently occurred during at least a proportion of the cycles characterized by short postswelling phases, only gradually did the secretion of progesterone become sufficient to effect rapid detumescence of the perineum and to support pregnancy.

The initial fecundity of women during the first 2 years after marriage at the ages of 15 to 19 is less than that of women married between the ages of 20 and 24 years (Table 1.4). Moreover,

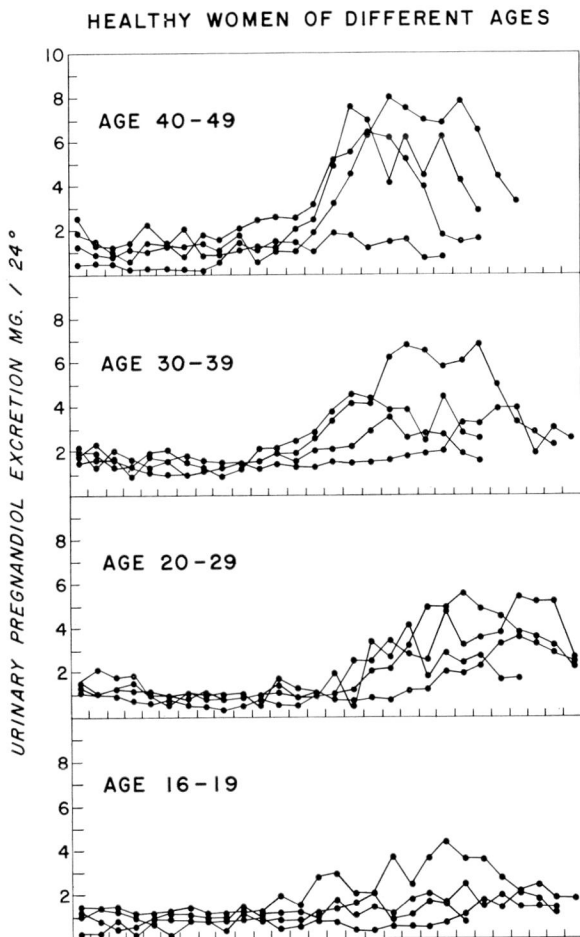

Fig. 1.6. The day-by-day excretion of pregnandiol in the urine of four normal women in each of four age groups. From Klopper.[8]

the average length and weight of children born to mothers ranging in age from 25 to 29 years is greater than that of infants born to younger women (Table 1.5). In rodents, what may be comparable observations are clearly related to the intensity of gonadotropic stimulation. Both the number of the corpora lutea[9] and the average number of young born[7] are greater in the second litter than in the first.

TABLE 1.3

The Reproductive Performance of Adolescent Chimpanzees Mated at Two Different Stages of Sexual Maturation*

Stage of Development at which Mating Permitted	Proportion of Fertile Matings	Proportion of Abortions within 100 Days of Conception
Postswelling phase of 8 days or less	11/78 (14%)	4/11 (36%)
Postswelling phase longer than 8 days	53/177 (30%)	9/51 (18%)

* Conception and abortion rates within 100 days of conception in adolescent chimpanzees permitted to mate at different stages of sexual development. (The normal length of pregnancy in the chimpanzee is 226 days). From Young and Yerkes.[19]

TABLE 1.4

The Initial Fecundity of Newly Married Women of Different Ages*

Ages of Wives Newly Married	Delivering During the First Two Years
	%
15–19	43.7
20–24	90.5
25–29	75.8
30–34	62.9
35–39	41.0
40–44	15.5
45–49	4.4

* The effect of the wife's age upon her fecundity during the first 2 years of marriage. From Duncan.[5]

TABLE 1.5

The Effect of Maternal Age Upon Infant Size*

Age of Mother	Average Length	Average Weight
	in.	lb., oz
15–19	19.007	6, 15.7
20–24	19.168	7, 3.5
25–29	19.355	7, 6.5
30–34	19.229	7, 4.3
35–39	18.899	7, 4.4
40–44	18.910	7, 2.5
45–49	18.166	6, 14.7

* The average length and weight of children born to mothers of different ages. From Duncan.[5]

In early puberty, therefore, "adolescent sterility" appears to reflect an LH deficiency so severe as to preclude ovulation; at a later stage, the quantity of LH released suffices to induce ovulation but fails to effect mature corpus luteum formation and/or function. Whether the LH deficiency is a consequence of inadequate pituitary secretion or of a deficiency of the hypothalamic LH releasing factor remains to be determined.

Both neonatal and maternal mortality and the proportion of stillbirths is higher in adolescent primiparas than in older women. However, it is not clear whether immaturity *per se* increases the propensity to complications since adolescent patients have often received inadequate prenatal care. Of the 24 mice mentioned previously which conceived at the first estrus, 7 died during parturition. It may be that "adolescent sterility" subserves a protective function.

In conclusion, it is evident that only gradually does the adolescent attain peak reproductive efficiency. Just as the occurrence of the menarche, a dramatic marker on the path of sexual maturation, does not necessarily connote fertility, so ovulation and the earliest conceptions do not imply the achievement of full reproductive competence. In a biological sense, adolescence is less a flowering than a slow blooming and requires the lapse of more than a decade.

REFERENCES

1. Brown, J. B.: Urinary excretion of oestrogens during the menstrual cycle. Lancet, *1:* 320, 1955.
2. Brown, P. S.: Human urinary gonadotrophins. I. In relation to puberty. J. Endocrinol., *17:* 329, 1958.
3. Collett, M. E., Wertenberger, G. E., and Fiske, V. M.: The effect of age upon the pattern of the menstrual cycle. Fertil. & Steril., *5:* 437, 1954.
4. Cooperman, N. R.: The relationship of adolescent menstruation to body temperature and sterility. Am. J. Obst. & Gynec., *57:* 701, 1949.
5. Duncan, J. M.: *Fertility, Fecundity and Related Topics*. Adam and Charles Black, Edinburgh, 1871.
6. Fitschen, W., and Clayton, B. E.: Urinary excretion of gonadotrophins with particular reference to children. Arch. Dis. Childhood, *40:* 16, 1965.

7. King, H. D.: Litter production and the sex ratio in various strains of rats. Anat. Rec., *27:* 337, 1924.
8. Klopper, A. I.: The excretion of pregnanediol during the normal menstrual cycle. J. Obst. & Gynaec. Brit. Emp., *64:* 504, 1957.
9. MacDonald, E. C., and Lord, E. M.: Number of corpora lutea in successive mouse pregnancies. Anat. Rec., *31:* 131, 1925.
10. McArthur, J. W.: Functional disorders of menstruation in adolescence. New England J. Med., *249:* 361, 1953.
11. McArthur, J. W.: Adolescent menstrual disorders. In *Progress in Gynecology*, Vol. 3, p. 153. Grune and Stratton, Inc., New York, 1957.
12. McArthur, J. W., Ingersoll, F. M., and Worcester, J.: Urinary excretion of interstitial-cell and follicle-stimulating hormone activity by women with diseases of the reproductive system. J. Clin. Endocrinol., *18:* 1202, 1958.
13. Mirskaia, L., and Crew, F. A. E.: Maturity in the female mouse. Proc. Roy. Soc. Edinburgh, *50:* 179, 1930.
14. Nathanson, I. T., Towne, L. E., and Aub, J. C.: Normal excretion of sex hormones in childhood. Endocrinology, *28:* 851, 1941.
15. Persson. Data published by Diczfalusy, E., and Lauritzen, C.: *Oestrogene beim Menschen*. Springer-Verlag, Kiel, 1961.
16. Pinkerton, J. H. M.: Oestrogen production in the immature human ovary (observations based upon histochemical studies). J. Obst. & Gynaec. Brit. Emp., *66:* 820, 1959.
17. Savard, K., Marsh, J. M., and Rice, B. F.: Gonadotropins and ovarian steroidogenesis. In *Recent Progress in Hormone Research*, Vol. 21, p. 285. Academic Press, Inc., New York, 1965.
18. Talbot, N. B., Sobel, E. H., McArthur, J. W., and Crawford, J. D.: *Functional Endocrinology from Birth through Adolescence*. Harvard University Press, Cambridge, Mass., 1954.
19. Young, W. C., and Yerkes, R. M.: Factors influencing the reproductive cycle in the chimpanzee; the period of adolescent sterility and related problems. Endocrinology, *33:* 121, 1943.

2

The Biochemistry of Steroids and Hormones

Charles W. Lloyd, M.D.

Today, I plan to talk to you about biochemistry as I, as a clinician, understand it. I'm going to talk about endocrine regulation and the interrelationships of the endocrine system.

The steroid secreting glands—the ovary, testis, and adrenal—make hormones which are released into blood, in general, in free form, although there is evidence that, at least in the adrenal, the material may be released as a sulfate. The steroid is bound for transport in blood by plasma proteins. In this form it is carried to the liver, which is the primary site of clearance. I'm speaking about metabolic clearance and not renal clearance alone. This gets rid of steroids from the blood and occurs primarily in the liver. The rate at which the steroids are removed tends in general to be related to the tightness of binding to the proteins. For example, cortisol is bound quite tightly to its transporting protein whereas aldosterone is bound very loosely. The clearance of aldosterone is about 10 times that of cortisol and correlates quite nicely with the tightness of binding. In the liver, the steroids are not only removed and degraded to less potent forms, they are conjugated with sulfates or glucuronides. This makes them water soluble, which increases the rate with which they can be excreted. They are also changed into other steroids that haven't, as yet, been studied much. People in my lab call these the unpopular steroids because they are not the ones that we hear about most. These may be of considerable significance in modifying actions of other hormones and in feedback to the hypothalamus which regulates secretion of the trophic hormones. One illustration of this is the possibility that the 6-hydroxycortisol, which is an excretory product of the adrenal hormone and doesn't have any known effect in comparison with the usual adrenal steroids, may actually have an effect in inhibiting these materials. Similarly, estriol under certain conditions can inhibit the action of the other estrogens. It is possible that these things not only inhibit peripherally but that they also inhibit the action of the primary secretory product of the gland at the hypothalamic centers that regulate the trophic hormones.

I think I'll start now with the more or less classical schemes of the way the steroids are made. In the adrenal, starting with acetate, there are various substances converted to cholesterol. From cholesterol, pregnenolone and progesterone are synthesized and from these one gets the usual adrenal steroids. Adrenocorticotropic hormone (ACTH) probably acts in a number of places. One place it acts is in the conversion of cholesterol to pregnenolone. Beginning with acetate one builds up cholesterol and from cholesterol one can go on through pregnenolone and progesterone, which are common pathways in all of the steroids, to the androgens and estrogens as well as to the adrenal steroids.

Another pathway is now beginning to be of considerable interest, that I will mention for completeness. It may very well not only be cholesterol itself that is an intermediate but also cholesterol sulfate, and cholesterol sulfate may end up as an androgen and particularly a corticosteroid. The reason I mention this is that, as you will see later on, I'll have to talk to you a little bit about some techniques by which these schemes have been worked up. It's quite possible that conditions of study of these things might favor a certain pathway which might be very important *in vivo*.

Let us consider the general scheme of both adrenal and ovarian synthesis of sex steroids from cholesterol. The important points here are simply these: Cholesterol goes to pregnenolone and progesterone, the common pathway. From these are formed the androgens, mostly androstenedione, but also testosterone. The production of testosterone involves the conversion of androstenedione to testosterone. And it is from these androgens that the estrogens ultimately are made. This is not only true in the adrenal and the ovary, but also in the testicle.

It is important to re-emphasize that starting with progesterone one goes through androstenedione and ends up with testosterone.

Now that the steroids are made, it is necessary to get rid of them. A major site of conversion is the liver. The rate of clearance is dependent on the tightness of binding to plasma protein. Cortisol, which is tightly bound, is cleared much less than aldosterone, which is loosely bound.

Cortisol is first saturated to form the tetrahydrocortisol in the liver. This is excreted as such or its conjugate. It has to be saturated in ring A before it can be conjugated. This is the defect in cirrhosis. When cortisol is given to a cirrhotic, he doesn't form the conjugate, tetrahydrocortisol glucuronide, as well as the normal individual. The reason is not that he can't hook the glucuronide on, but that he can't saturate the ring. This is one of the primary forms in which the cortisol is excreted. Also the side chain can be cleaved, resulting in 17-ketosteroids, these particular 17-ketosteroids retaining the oxygen function at the 11th carbon.

There are a number of metabolites of the various adrenal steroids. Among these are tetrahydrocortisol and tetrahydrocortisone with ring A saturated and the 17-ketosteroids which retain the oxygen at 11. From the other adrenal steroids, there are various 17-ketosteroids. In general, the 17-ketosteroids tend to reflect adrenal function because, although testosterone is excreted as a 17-ketosteroid, so are many other adrenal steroids. These other adrenal steroids can go to etiocholanolone and androstenedione. As I'll point out a little later, the amount of 17-ketosteroids that can come from testosterone is so small, because the amount of testosterone made is so small, that it really does not add much to the total urinary 17-ketosteroids.

Let's consider the kind of scheme one would expect for estrogens. The androgens (androstenedione and testosterone) form estradiol and estrone, which are more or less interconvertible. Probably in the liver they are degraded to various estrogens, the principal one being estriol. And you'll remember from Dr. McArthur's discussion of Brown's data that estriol is present in the largest amount in the urine when estradiol and estrone are secreted by the steroid producing organ or when they are given parenterally.

I'd like to digress for a moment to discuss a very interesting compound that may have a lot of clinical significance (at least to the rabbit, from which it comes). Actually, it gives a clue concerning some possible factors in estrogen action. This is a compound that Dr. Donald Lane, who works in our institution, has isolated from rabbit urine. It is one of the principal metabolites of estrogen that are in the urine of the rabbit. This compound is estradiol with the glucuronide at C-3, and an acetyl glucosamine at C-17. Structurally this compound is exactly similar to the mucopolysaccharides of the uterus. Is it possible that the body in some way hooks these groups on to make this estrogen nucleus more acceptable to the uterus? May it be, in other words, that this is a way that the estrogen gets into the uterus? As has been clearly shown, particularly by the work of Jenson, estrogen, particularly estradiol, does concentrate in the uterus. It may be that in this way it gets there.

Here is another interesting compound of Dr. Lane's. This substance points out the problems that are involved in assaying what is going on as far as estrogen is concerned by the urinary bio-assay or by the chemical assay. Norethynodrel, the gestogen in Enovid, is excreted as about 30 per cent in this particular form. A small amount of it goes out as ethinyl estradiol. There are reports that when norethynodrel is given to humans more estrogenic activity than would be expected in the urine results. It may be coming from degradation to ethinyl estradiol which is an extremely potent estrogen. The principal product is not of itself estrogenic but a very potent compound in potentiating estrogen. If you give an estrogen to an animal and add this to it, it will markedly enhance estrogenic activity. So that it may very well be that when one does a bio-assay of estrogen, one can be fooled by the presence of these potentiators. On the other hand, it is quite possible that when one measures the estrogen chemically, one could miss this, and therefore miss the biological activity. This is why I believe that in the future when we do get the best possible chemical methods, we're also going to have to develop better bio-assay methods. What we're really interested in is what hormones do in the organism, not what numbers one can get from the chemicals in urine.

I'd like to discuss very quickly the ways in which one gets information about metabolism and synthesis of the steroids in the human. As I've indicated, one can get a lot of information from substances in the urine, and one can give a compound and see what metabolites come out in the urine. Most of this information has been obtained by giving exogenous steroids. One can try to measure the steroids in blood, for example, the corticosteroids. This does not tell what is made but gives a crude idea of how much is made; there is some correlation between the secretion rate and the levels in blood.

Other techniques of studying the steroid production involve methods for estimation of production rates. If one wants to know how much of X steroid is made, X steroid or a unique metabolite of X steroid can be measured in the urine. The individual is given radioisotope labeled X steroid in a tracer amount. The urine is collected for three or four days, and the amount of the material there that is not labeled, in other words, the amount that is cold, that comes from what the individual has made, is measured. The amount that is labeled is also measured. These data are expressed as a fraction. Since how much was given is known, from this fraction the denominator, or how much the individual made, can be calculated. The trouble with this is that a unique metabolite that can come from nothing else must be used. For example, in the male, testosterone glucuronide, which is a principal excretion form of testosterone, seems to come only from testosterone. There is little or no androstenedione made in the male. In the female, however, the evidence is that there is a lot of androstenedione made by the ovary. Very little, if any, testosterone is made by the ovary. As Tate has now deduced, most of the testosterone in the human plasma comes from conversion of androstenedione made by the ovary. It is confusing that androstenedione can go to the liver and there be converted directly to testosterone glucuronide. It is not converted into testosterone which is secreted and then converted to the glucuronide. Then there is excretion of a lot of testosterone glucuronide by the female that does not reflect testosterone secretion at all. So there must be some recalculating of production rates by this particular method.

Another method, called the urinary production rate method, measures production rates, the amount formed in the individual. This method uses the same principle, but by infusing the labeled steroid intravenously at a constant rate for a three- or four-hour period. This represents a kind of secretion of the labeled steroid. One also measures the unlabeled steroid at various intervals during this time. Measured amounts of both the labeled and unlabeled steroid are expressed as a fraction. If the unlabeled steroid increases in proportion to the labeled, more steroid is being made; if it decreases, less is secreted. From this test some very meaningful data can be obtained.

The last way, from which a lot of information has been obtained, is by incubation *in vitro* of various endocrine glands. The difficulty with this is (1) extrapolating from a test tube what's happening in the total organism, and (2) comparing data from different laboratories. The reason that data don't agree seems to be that different incubation techniques are used and that the conditions are somehow different and give different yields of different steroids. It is also very important that the structures that are being incubated be identified. For instance, there are studies (I know of one) in which it is claimed that a particular fraction, microsomes for example, was incubated when this wasn't really the case. The conditons that are used, such as a particular starting substance, cofactors, and so on can change the pathway.

Similarly, the way in which the product is identified is very important. It must be known that the substance a scientist is talking about is what he thinks it is. This involves a number of meticulous chemical procedures. I stress this because there are many reports of finding particular substance that have not been really identified. Similarly, when one tries to quantitate the substances, one must recognize that these are not very efficient processes and there are large losses. One way to estimate losses is to add a marker; that is, if we're looking for estrone, we add a marked estrone. If we've incubated with a tritiated compound, we add C-14 estrone. The amount of the C-14 estrone added in the beginning is known; when this manipulation is completed the amount left is known; from this some idea of the recoveries can be gotten. Finally, it is necessary to remember that one cannot extrapolate from the test tube to the whole animal.

I want to go on to the question of androgens. Dr. McArthur presented what's known about the process of the menarche and the regulatory mechanism in humans. I think another area in which a tremendous amount of work must be done is concerned with the ways that steroids act in producing sexual maturation. Dr. Noumura, who has been working with us, has worked out a technique for sexing the fetuses of rats. He can tell a difference at $13\frac{1}{2}$ days between male and female gonads. The rat's gestation period is $21\frac{1}{2}$ days. At $13\frac{1}{2}$ days, Dr. Noumura has been able to collect testicles and ovaries, incubate them, and find out what they make. They don't make much of anything at $13\frac{1}{2}$ days, but by $14\frac{1}{2}$ days they're active, and by $15\frac{1}{2}$ days they make lots of testosterone and androstenedione. The fetal ovary doesn't make much of anything. By the time of birth, the testis makes very large amounts of androgen. The fetal testis is a much more efficient testosterone synthesizer than that of older animals. The older animal makes other steroids such as estrogens.

It is the androgen of the fetus that produces Wolffian differentiation. In the absence of androgen, no differentiation as a male occurs but the Müllerian system fuses. The castrated fetus of either sex has differentiation of the Müllerian system. It also is the presence of androgen that differentiates the hypothalamus. In the rat, at least, the newborn animal has a female hypothalamus; that is, the hypothalamus is capable of causing cyclic release of gonadotropin. If androgen doesn't alter this, the male hypothalamus retains this cyclicity. It does so right through life if the testis is removed at birth. If the animal is castrated at birth and at 200 days ovaries are put in, those ovaries will ovulate. On the other hand, if one gives testosterone to a newborn female animal, that animal never cycles; it has the lack of cyclicity of the male. I don't know why this doesn't happen in the fetus where there is much testosterone being made. It looks as though it's not getting to the hypothalamus, or if it gets there, something blocks its effects. There are some studies by Kimel and Dorfman (and we've confirmed and extended them) which indicate that progesterone given at the same time as testosterone to immature female animals will prevent this effect of androgen on the hypothalamus.

I don't know how busy the testes of the immature child are. I know that the gonads of the animal, long before adolescence, make more hormone than we would think, and I think the same thing applies to humans. One's ideas about when adolescence begins are necessarily very vague because I'm not sure adolescence ever begins. We may be having it all the time. In other words, from birth there may be small amounts of steroid production which increase later in life. Certainly oophorectomy of a very young rat will result in a noticeably smaller uterus in the middle of its pre-adolescence, that is, when the animal is 18 days of age. These animals have vaginal opening at about 40 days. If the ovaries of these animals are removed very early in life, by 18 or 20 days, the uterus is about half the size of that of a normal animal. This ovary makes estrogen early in life.

Now, I want to talk about some data from adults concerning androgens. We've measured testosterone in blood by techniques that are complicated but accurate. There's a quite narrow range of testosterone in normal women. The only time one finds higher values, values above one standard deviation above the mean, is at ovulation or later. Clinically, I think this is of importance because this may very well explain the premenstrual acne that occurs in so many individuals. This fits in with what one would predict from the production of estrogen, because the estrogen level, too, would reach a peak at ovulation and would be higher during the luteal phase than it was during the follicular phase.

There is no correlation between the testosterone in blood and urinary 17-ketosteroids in the normal individual. Because there's so little testosterone made (about half a milligram is the production rate per day in the woman) it just couldn't influence the 17-ketosteroids.

However, in women who are hirsute there is a correlation. The reason seems to be that the 17-ketosteroids reflect over-all activity of the adrenal. During increased activity of this type of producing all kinds of subject, testosterone is made, so there is a correlation between urinary ketosteroids and plasma testosterone. In the case of a young woman, 19 years of age, who had untreated congenital adrenal hyperplasia, there was a good correlation, because the adrenal was making all kinds of things besides testosterone and these things are reflected in the urinary ketosteroids. Without therapy, she has 17-ketosteroids of 90 mg. or so; a 24-hour plasma testosterone value that is in the male range, 10 times the normal female levels. When we gave her corticosteroids, they both suppressed.

We've done a study of women with various kinds of hirsutism. I'll show you some of the correlations. We gave these women ACTH and studied plasma testosterone and urinary ketosteroids before and after treatment; we suppressed the adrenal with dexamethazone and then we gave the women chorionic gonadotropin in an attempt to stimulate the ovary and studied the same parameters.

The urinary 17-ketosteroids don't correlate with the hirsutism. The plasma testosterones are elevated in all patients who have hirsutism.

When ACTH is given, one sees an increase in urinary 17-ketosteroids in normal women, and about the same amount in women with the polycystic ovaries. Those women who have idiopathic hirsutism have tremendously increased 17-ketosteroids just as they have markedly increased response in the plasma testosterone. Neither women with the polycystic ovary nor normal women have an appreciable increase in plasma testosterone when the adrenal is stimulated.

When the adrenal is inhibited, the 17-ketosteroids are nicely suppressed in both the normal women and the women who have idiopathic hirsutism, but in patients with polycystic ovaries the 17-ketosteroids don't go down. Similarly, the subjects with idiopathic hirsutism have a considerably greater decrease in plasma testosterone.

When one has primarily a problem with the ovary, as with the polycystic ovary, and chorionic gonadotropin is given, there is a greater increase in the 17-ketosteroids and in the plasma testosterone than in other subjects.

There may be considerable difference in responsiveness to hormones. As you know, the Orientals don't have nearly as much body hair as Caucasians. I'm told that in Japan some gynecologists have many requests to grow more body hair on Japanese women by giving testosterone. That made me think that maybe they have lower testosterone levels. Dr. Kobyashi, who worked with us last year, did a study of plasma testosterone and urinary

17-ketosteroids of Japanese and Caucasians living in Massachusetts. To make sure there was not any environmental component, we got a number of plasmas and urines from Tokyo. There is no difference in plasma testosterones in women or men of either race. There are about two-thirds of the urinary 17-ketosteroids in both Japanese males and females compared to Caucasians. This ratio is expressed in terms of body surface, so it isn't just a matter of body mass. The Japanese have a difference in something. That is mirrored in 17-ketosteroids but not the plasma testosterone. This type of evidence makes me think that there is something besides testosterone that may influence androgenicity.

Many patients have evidence that psychological factors not only influence the menstrual cycle but also increase androgenicity. Some years ago some remarks of mine to this effect appeared in the *Ladies Home Journal*. I said that I had seen an increase in body hair occurring in women who had been through a severe psychological stress. I illustrated this by the history of the first patient who pointed this out to me, a girl whose father had committed suicide after he'd been indicted for embezzlement. She had then gotten involved sexually with a boy while she was in college and had a great deal of guilt about this. The boy went off to war; she went into an anxiety state, and within about two or three months she began to grow a lot of hair. A cartoon showing a young lady reading a letter breaking off her engagement and growing a beard was printed in the *Ladies Home Journal*. I had over 100 letters from ladies all over the United States saying, in essence, "Doctor, I discovered my husband's got a popsy down the street somewhere and I'm growing a beard." This is a pretty good testimonial to me that there is something evoked by psychological stress that plays a role. We've been doing some studies to see whether it could be that the catecholamines that might be evoked by psychological stress could have an effect here.

We've measured production rates of cortisol and of testosterone by the plasma method I described. A constant rate of the labeled steroid is given; then the dilution of this by the unlabeled steroid is measured throughout. We've looked for a change produced by epinephrine and have found that cortisol production rate increases in normal males and hirsute women but not in normal women. In males, testosterone production is decreased.

There seem to be various things that can influence the physiological effectiveness of a steroid. For example, the seminal vesicular weight of castrate animals was measured. Some rats were given testosterone, others the same amount of testosterone with cortisol in addition. Both the seminal vesicles and the prostates were markedly increased when cortisol was given in addition to testosterone. Cortisol in some way enhances the activity of the androgen. In other words, testosterone isn't the only thing that may influence androgenicity.

Let's discuss ovarian steroid synthesis for a moment. Savard has studied the *in vitro* production of various steroids by different parts of the ovaries. The cow corpus luteum makes only the gestogens. The human corpus luteum makes not only the gestogens but a little bit of androgen and quite a lot of estrogen. The human follicle makes the gestogens, some androgen, but it concentrates on making estrogens. The stroma tends to concentrate on making the androgens. It makes some estrogen, but less.

I'd like to close by discussing the way in which regulation of an organ can influence its production of steroids. If a normal female rat is given testosterone when it is 5 days of age, a curious thing happens. As a result of this androgen early in life, the animal has slight sexual precocity. It never has estrous cycles, and it eventually develops a cystic ovary with a fair increase in the amount of interstitial material. A similar ovary develops when this animal is exposed to constant light. After exposure to light for a few weeks, she fails to cycle anymore, and she develops ovaries that have a marked increase in interstitial areas without corpora lutea.

We've measured the pituitary gonadotropins of the animals that received testosterone. Early in life (15 days of age) a difference can be shown. The total gonadotropin is lower in the testosterone treated animal. In the normal animal, there is a very high level before puberty and a rapid drop at puberty, just before vaginal opening; then it would cycle. In the testosterone animal, it follows about the same pattern as the male, and it doesn't cycle. Similarly, luteinizing hormone of the testosterone animal is lower throughout life.

The crux of this matter is what the ovaries of these animals can make. Ovaries of normal animals incubated with progesterone make so little androgen that it can't be detected. They make an amount of estrogen that Dr. Judith Weisz, who has done these studies in our laboratory, can detect. Animals that have been given testosterone have ovaries that make enormous amounts of both estrogens and androgens.

The point is this. This is a reversible process which we have produced in normal animals. They secrete large amounts of estrogen and androgen. If the ovaries are taken out of these testosterone treated animals and implanted in normal animals, these animals will begin to ovulate and in a month the ovaries are biosynthetically right back to normal. We have produced what could be called enzymatic defects in animals affecting the regulatory mechanism. It is our belief that this is the same thing that happens in women who have polycystic ovaries. I believe that this syndrome is probably an acquired one, that there is not an inborn error of metabolism, an inborn synthetic defect. We have been able to show very high estrogen, as well as androgen, production in the polycystic ovaries of the human by these same techniques. We think that in the human there is some kind of aberration in hypothalamic regulation of gonadotropin that secondarily produces this defect in ovarian synthesis, a situation similar to what we have in these rats. In other words, this is an acquired defect that could be convertible back to the normal if we knew how to produce the right regulation.

3

The Identification of Sex Hormones by Chemical and Biological Assays

Joseph W. Goldzieher, M.D.

After you've been exposed to two hours of information packed lecturing, I find myself at a tremendous disadvantage—particularly so, because it is not my purpose to come before you with methodological details since you are not going to be doing hormone assays yourselves in the laboratory. My purpose is, perhaps, to give you a basis for individual discrimination when someone from a laboratory presents you with a number, a numerical value for some test. One's instinctive reaction is to take this as some sort of God-given figure which has a precision out to as many decimals as the person in the laboratory cared to put down. Further, my topic, "Sex Hormones," is really a very difficult one to delineate. The question in my mind is what do we mean by "sex hormones"? Consider a very schematic representation of things you've already heard today. The over-all sexual cycle involves the hypothalamus, including the preoptic center which probably introduces the rhythm into the estrus cycle of the rat and probably analogously the rhythm into the primate menstrual cycle. Then there are other hypothalamic centers, the ventromedial and the arcuate nuclei, which produce polypeptide hormones which in turn influence the pituitary; the pituitary in turn puts out other protein hormones or polypeptides (gonadotropins) and they stimulate the ovary to put out estrogens, testosterone or other androgens, and progestational compounds. So which of all of these am I to talk about methodologically in an hour? The matter simplifies itself considerably because we have very little information at the present time on the hypothalamic factors. Most current work is concerned with establishing their existence and perhaps their identity. And for our purposes, I think we can omit this area from the discussion.

However, when it comes to gonadotropins, as you've already heard from Dr. McArthur, there is a great deal of information available. Before we go into this, we must define what we require of a biological test, and how we are to evaluate it critically. The four great parameters, the criteria for any assay, bio-assay, or chemical assay, are these: accuracy, precision, sensitivity, and specificity. Until these are clearly specified, we do not know what a test is telling us. Accuracy means how close to the "real value" is the answer of our test. Precision or reproducibility is, if we do a bio-assay, the confidence limit of that bio-assay; if we do a chemical assay, the extent to which the value is good, the precision of duplicates, and so forth. Sensitivity, which we'll talk about repeatedly later on, is that value which we can distinguish from zero with a certain degree of confidence. And, finally, specificity means how we can discriminate that which we measure from all other spurious substances which seem to give us the same endpoint. When we apply this to the problem of gonadotropins, we have considerable difficulty, because gonadotropins are measured with bio-assays and the precision of bio-assays is far from what one would like. It is all too common, in our clinical laboratories, to assay total gonadotropins by the so-called Klinefelter assay; this is the result of weighing two, or four, or six ovaries; the primitiveness of this assay to a professional bio-assayist is beyond description. Yet a great deal of the endocrine literature that one reads today is based on mouse ovarian weights based on two or four mice. As a matter of fact, except for Johnson, who claims that his total gonadotropin method can reliably detect gonadotropins in the normal female or the normal male, most workers in the gonadotropin field feel that you cannot distinguish the values obtained under normal circumstances from zero. There we have, as you see, a great problem in sensitivity.

Now consider the gonadotropin excretion of a postmenopausal woman as shown by Eugenia Rosenberg's work; it illustrates the great day-to-day variation of urinary gonadotropins which one would think would remain at a fairly constant level. Thus, one must ask oneself: If I collect a 24-hour urine and get a value, what does that value mean? Quite clearly it means nothing, because one can get either a highly elevated "postmenopausal" level or a zero level in the same woman, depending on the day the urine is collected. If one wants to get a meaningful value from an individual such as this, one must pool at least a week's urine and do the gonadotropin determination in a reliable fashion, on a suitable number of animals, with a good experimental bio-assay design. Then one might arrive at a number which has a ±20 per cent confidence limit.

Another thing which concerns us is the fact that most of the assays which have been reported until very recently measure *total* gonadotropin. There is no such thing as "total gonadotropin." Gonadotropins are, at least in man, of two kinds, as you heard, follicle-stimulating hormone (FSH) and luteinizing hormone (LH). And since, as you have seen, there is enormous variation in the ratio of one to the other in the normal menstrual cycle, what one measures in a random urine in terms of qualitative activity is very questionable. The best proof of this is, for example, in studies on adult women receiving oral contraceptives. John Loraine and his group repeatedly find "normal" values for urinary gonadotropins in women taking various oral contraceptives. This is clearly at variance with the facts, because these women do not ovulate and histologically their ovaries are quiescent. When selective FSH and LH assays are done, it is found that estrogens do one thing to FSH and LH, progestational compounds do another thing to FSH and LH, and a combination does still a third thing to FSH and LH. None of this is seen with a so-called total gonadotropin determination. Gradually people are leaning more and more to specific assays for FSH and LH. This is an area for the professional bio-assayist which over the years has generated a great deal of debate, and I don't propose to get myself involved in whether one method is more reliable than another. Usually, the Steelman-Pohley assay is accepted for FSH determinations, and for LH the ovarian ascorbic acid depletion test is probably the most sensitive and the most useful. Dr. Stevens at Ohio State, for example, can perform ovarian ascorbic acid tests on 48- and sometimes 24-hour urines throughout the cycle. Thus, sensitivity is getting to be in the range where meaningful data can be obtained. There has been a great deal of talk about the phenomenal sensitivity of the ovarian cholesterol assay; in the hands of most people it has not been working satisfactorily. Finally, there is some promise that immunological methods, immuno-assays for FSH and LH will be developed. The Boston Group in particular has been working very hard on immuno-assays. Of course, the big problem is to have immunochemically pure FSH and LH. Our best LH preparations still cross-react with chorionic gonadotropins and no FSH made today is absolutely free of contaminants. This is about the state of the art as far as bio-assays of gonadotropins are concerned.

We might make some other comments about bio-assay in general. In a bio-assay we are using the response of an animal of a species other than the human, and there are some large and important questions that this raises. For example, is the physiology of that test animal comparable to the physiology of man, so that the results are meaningful? This is a very serious question. Take for example, the rat. It requires FSH, LH, *and prolactin* to bring about hormone secretion by the ovary; whereas, it takes only FSH and LH in the human, and prolactin is not required. Therefore, there is a fundamental difference in the physiology of the entire system. Whether rat data can be related, except perhaps in the broadest sense, to human data becomes a debatable question. Another classical example is a drug by the name of clomiphene. Clomiphene was originally tested in rodents and found to be an excellent antifertility drug—100% effective. In man, as you all know, it is used to *promote* ovulation in anovulatory women.

What about the sensitivity of the animal as related to sensitivity in man? One of the most useful tests for measuring the gonadotropin inhibiting power of estrogens, for example, is a preparation known as the parabiotic rat. In the parabiotic rat, estrone is many, many times more potent than ethyl estradiol so far as inhibiting the pituitary goes. In the human, it is exactly the reverse. When one does experiments on pituitary inhibition in the parabiotic rat, what do they mean in terms of human physiology, when we get the diametrically opposite results with test compounds? These are very important questions. In the bio-assay of the steroidal sex hormones, the test tissues are the seminal vesicles, the levator ani, the ventral prostate, and so on. If one were to take time to delve into the literature, one would be staggered by the lack of information correlating any parallelism between these assays and androgenicity in man. As a matter of fact, one of the most depressing enterprises I have undertaken was to try to find good bio-assay data in man of the androgenicity of some very important compounds. In man two indices of some value (and often they are quite neglected) are the volume of the seminal fluid, an excellent rough indicator of androgenic activity in the male, and, as Hamilton showed many years ago, the rate of growth of axillary hair. These are both exceedingly crude bio-assays, but at least they are in the species in which we are interested.

With estrogens one would think that one is in a better position, because the vaginal smear or the endometrial biopsy have been used widely in animals and in man, and we like to equate the cornification or the karyopyknotic index of the vaginal smear with estrogen output. The troubles with this bio-assay are manyfold. The end organ, the vaginal epithelium, is certainly the most sensitive of all the structures responding to estrogen, but it is not exclusively sensitive to estrogen. It can be opposed. For instance, if one were to give simultaneously testosterone along with estrogen, one would get an entirely false idea of how much estrogen had been given to that experimental animal because the testosterone (or many other steroids) opposes at the site of the target organ the biological effect seen as "estrogenic activity." The converse of this is augmentation, as you have already seen from some of the examples given by Dr. Lloyd. And what is worse, the Japanese have shown that a castrate mouse of a certain species will cornify its vaginal epithelium without any estrogen at all. So one cannot take these endpoints at their face value. I think one of the greatest mistakes we make in clinical medicine is to say that a person is not *producing any estrogen* when we see an "atrophic" or a "hypo-estrogenic" vaginal smear. All we can say—and it is a very important distinction

—is that *at this target organ* an estrogenic effect is or is not seen. Whether estrogen is produced or opposed is something else again.

When we come to the progestational compounds, one would again hope for simplicity. Progesterone is progesterone, so all one has to measure is some biological activity of progesterone and presto, we have a bio-assay. However, there are a variety of actions of progesterone and bio-assays have been constructed on the basis of each one. And, unfortunately, depending on the progestational compound taken, these various parameters do not run parallel. For example, there are some compounds which have very powerful endometrial activity and no pregnancy maintenance activity. Some are very powerful in pituitary blockage but very weak in some other effect. A progestin is not a simple thing. Progestational activity is a complex of activities; one must first decide which biological parameter of progestational activity is of interest, and then one must design the bio-assay accordingly. In very rough terms, the endometropic activity (as the Clauberg assay in the rat) and the endometrial carbonic anhydrase activity parallel in very rough fashion the endometrial activity in man. We have found fairly good agreement between Clauberg potency and potency in terms of progestational changes in the estrogen primed human endometrium. So, very briefly, this presents a rather iconoclastic view of the problems which we face with bioassay of these hormones.

Let us turn to chemical assays of steroid hormones in the hope that here at least we have nice definable compounds that we can isolate and measure and from which we can get numerical values with a good confidence limit. Alas, it isn't quite that simple. What is it that we are going to assay? If we are interested in androgenic activity, there is, as you've already heard, no single compound that possesses all the biological activity that we're after. We may have a pure compound but it may not be the only compound; indeed, it may not even be the most interesting compound. In fact, most of the time we don't even know which hormone accounts for the desired action. It was not until four or five years ago that we began to appreciate the importance of testosterone in the female as the agent responsible for many androgenic effects. For years we have worried about what is the adrenal androgen, and the debate still goes on. So, in spite of the fact that we can get a nice chemical determination for this steroid or that steroid, we haven't answered the basic question of what we want to assay.

Then come the other questions which Dr. Lloyd has already touched upon. In what form is this hormone active? How does the form that we measure correlate with the form which acts on the tissue to produce the effect that we are interested in clinically? If we measure some product or metabolite of that hormone, is it invariably a representative portion? And where do we measure it, since its concentration at the target cell is not measurable? Shall we measure it in blood? In blood we have problems. In blood there are active or inactive forms—free steroid and steroid which is bound to substances like transcortin or other proteins. The hormone may be conjugated to sulfuric or glucuronic acid, or it may be free. It may vary from hour to hour (as the diurnal variation of the adrenal steroids) or it may show week-to-week fluctuations or day-to-day fluctuations as, for example, the estrogens and progesterone compounds. So a single determination in blood gives us perhaps one frame of a motion picture. I grant that if you see one frame of a moving picture with 6000 people and a palace in it, it's probably Cecil B. DeMille, but that won't include the vast majority of movies that you're going to see. And the same will be true of a single measurement in blood. What about urine? A 24-hour urine collection has the great advantage that it is an integrated output over 24 hours and in that sense one has ironed out the rapid fluctuations which present a problem with determinations in blood. However, the urinary output depends on the transport mechanism in the blood, whether the hormones are tightly or loosely bound, and it also depends in certain disease states on the renal clearance. Is the measured material representative of the active material? This is sometimes a very sticky question indeed. If it is a metabolite, is it proportional under all conditions? We know, for example, in the case of the estrogens, that the estrone estradiol estriol ratio is substantially changed in patients with myocardial infarction. Why this is we do not know, but it is a fact. So, if we measure only 1 of the 3 major metabolites or 2 out of the whole 15 or so, are we really getting a representative estimate of what is being produced? It is for reasons such as these that the more dynamic tests which Dr. Lloyd touched on—the secretion rate, the metabolic clearance rate, and so on—have received great attention over the last few years.

Let us talk about the androgens. As you have already heard, the androgens come from two pathways, the Δ5 group from pregnenolone down to dehydroepiandrosterone and the Δ4 group from progesterone down to androstenedione and testosterone. They derive from the adrenal and from the gonads of *either* sex. Thus there are a variety of compounds which have androgenic activity: the testosterone-androstenedione pair, dehydroepiandrosterone and its sulfate (which are very different metabolically and probably also in terms of androgenic effectiveness), and finally a group which has an additional oxygen in position 11, the 11-oxy-17-ketosteroids, whose androgenic activity is still inadequately defined.

If one were to measure all these compounds or a single one, how reliable would be the estimate of androgenicity? Worse still, how do these compounds interact in terms of inhibition or augmentation to produce the ultimate clinical effect? If we recognize this problem and agree that for the moment it is insoluble, one might concentrate, for example, simply on testosterone and its estimation. One cannot measure testosterone from its metabolites, because both dehydroepiandrosterone and testosterone yield the same two metabolites, androsterone and etiocholanolone. These two, in turn, differ only in the orientation of a single *proton* at the 5-position in the molecule. Now, this may seem a trivial point, and of no interest to a clinician, but unfortunately it is not trivial. Androsterone is androgenic; etiocholanolone is not. The proportion of these two which is made from a given amount of dehydroepiandrosterone is influenced by other endocrine glands, particularly the thyroid. So, in thyroid deficiency, there will be a much higher proportion metabolized to androsterone than usual, and, therefore, for a given production of dehydroepiandrosterone there will be more peripheral androgenic activity than in the euthyroid individual. It has been postulated that this is the basis of so-called juvenile hypothyroid hirsutism. If one cannot measure the metabolites of testosterone because dehydroepiandrosterone also ends up in the same things, in much larger quantities, how about measuring testosterone in the urine itself? This is more easily said than done because the concentration of testosterone in the urine in males runs from about 0.05 to 0.17 mg. per day and in females runs from about 0.01 to 0.03 mg. per day, which are extremely small quantities. What is worse is that there are approximately equal amounts of another substance, *epi*testosterone, in the urine and this unrelated material is very difficult to separate from testosterone. Testosterone in plasma can be measured by very sophisticated laboratories, such as the laboratories of Dr. Lloyd, Dr. Simmer, and some others. Here one is dealing with fractions of micrograms per 100 ml. of plasma. This means that a precise method, sensitive enough to use small amounts of plasma, must detect nanograms of testosterone. This is very difficult to accomplish, but it is finally being done. The important thing about free testosterone, whether it is in the urine or in the plasma, is that testosterone is not a 17-ketosteroid. Therefore, no device which measures 17-ketosteroids will measure testosterone itself.

What about dehydroepiandrosterone, the major C-19 steroid produced by the adrenal? It is presumably moderately androgenic, although good bio-assays in humans have never been done. Is it androgenic perhaps because some of it is converted to testosterone? Studies with dehydroepiandrosterone have been complicated in the last few years by the discovery that it is produced by the adrenal not only as the free steroid but conjugated as the sulfate, and these two compounds are metabolically very different. For example, the half-life of the free compound is about 45 min., that of the sulfate about 9 hrs. These compounds, both free and sulfate, are partly broken down to androsterone and etiocholanolone in the urine and these three, D, A, and E* are of course 17-ketosteroids. There are other adrenal steroids, particularly 11β-hydroxyandrostenedione, which can arise either as such, in the adrenal, or from the cleavage of hydrocortisone. Its metabolites also appear in the urine as 17-ketosteroids. Thus, we come to a discussion of the 17-ketosteroids, what they mean, and how one measures them. Obviously, from what has been said, there are two groups of 17-ketosteroids, those with two oxygens (D, A, and E), and those with three oxygens, which come exclusively from the adrenal either *de novo* or by peripheral breakdown of hydrocortisone. Thus, a patient with Cushing's syndrome might have an elevated 17-ketosteroid value, but little of

---

* D, dehydroepiandrosterone; A, androsterone; E, etiocholanolone.

it might be D, A, or E, and most of it might be 11-oxy 17-ketosteroids; then one wouldn't know whether the ketosteroids came from the breakdown of all the cortisol or from more androgenic sources.

The 17-ketosteroids are excreted as two types of conjugates—sulfates and the glucuronides. The procedure for measuring 17-ketosteroids is to break these conjugates either by enzymatic hydrolysis or by cooking with acid. After more or less clean-up, purification of one kind or another, measurement is made by the familiar Zimmerman reaction. Unfortunately, the words "Zimmerman reaction" elicit little from the clinician except an act of faith, and if the report states that the excretion is 9.1 mg. per day, this is taken to mean exactly 9.1, not 9.0 or 9.2. In fact, the Zimmerman reaction is a highly sensitive, highly unspecific reaction for all sorts of ketones. Ordinary laboratory alcohol will give a beautiful Zimmerman reaction because there are aldehydes and ketones in it. *This* is the reaction on which one depends when it is reported that the 17-ketosteroid output is such-and-such.

In the old days, people were more careful with their 17-ketosteroid determinations and purified the urinary extract by a step called a Girard reaction. If this step is done, and if the total 17-ketosteroid value by a Girard reaction is compared to the value obtained by isolating all the 17-ketosteroids and adding them up, one obtains an exceedingly good correlation. When the 17-keto test became more popular, and demand increased, the clinical laboratory men obliged by making the method simpler and simpler, to turn out more of them, faster.

If one examines some of these newer clinical methods and assesses them against their true content of 17-ketosteroids, one should see the same correlation as with Girard purified extracts. In fact, with the ordinary 17-ketosteroid determination, the value obtained may be up to 80 per cent "chromogen" which is not 17-ketosteroids of adrenal or gonadal origin at all. It is amazing to me that 17-ketosteroid determinations correlate even as well as they do with other parameters such as dynamic tests by adrenocorticotropic hormone (ACTH) stimulation and dexamethasone suppression. Recognizing these problems, what can we do about them? There are methods available, either by thin layer chromatography or column chromatography whereby the steroids can be freed of all nonspecific material and then split into the 11-oxy and 11-desoxy ketosteroids, thus giving a much better picture of the nature of things. At least the 11-desoxys will give the sum total of D, testosterone, and androstenedione production and won't be clouded by the 11-oxys which come exclusively from the adrenal. Lately gas chromatography has become very popular. One can take a urinary extract, make a derivative of it, and squirt this into a gas chromatograph. It is a very useful tool for measuring 17-ketosteroids when somebody who knows what he is doing is using it. But many of the reports now in the clinical laboratory literature show an abysmal ignorance of the limitations of this method.

Now we come to the estrogens. The number of estrogens in the urine is staggering, and I call to your attention the fact that even by the Brown method (which is the one that is most widely used) only the three major ones are ever measured. In pregnancy 2-methoxyestrone may be exceedingly important. The 2-hydroxy and 2-methoxy estrogens are very important in the metabolism of tissues, for example, the prostate, the adrenal, and the kidney. Again we come to the famous question, if we measure only X out of a possible Y metabolite, how truly are we measuring the real estrogen production or activity?

There is a great range of variation of output of the three major estrogens in the normal cycle. Therefore, when estrogen levels vary as rapidly as they do, one has to ask oneself, what does a single urinary estrogen determination mean? Certainly in the normal, cycling woman it gives absolutely no information except that there is or is not estrogen at that time. One is not very likely to get much insight into follicle or corpus luteum activity without measuring the day-by-day curve of estrogen output.

With low levels of estrogen excretion, as in postmenopausal women or children, there is the problem of discrimination. With values this low, what does the value mean? Of the material which is measured by an allegedly specific reaction, how much is really estrogen? The only real comparison of the Kober method, the Brown method, and the isotope dilution method was one that was carried out by the Sloan-Kettering group, and the data are as follows: To two patients they gave intravenously 2000 μg. of estrogens and then compared the results by isotope dilution and by the Brown method; they agreed. In the one woman who was a castrate and hypophysectomized, in a single pooled urine there was reasonable agreement. On the basis of this one experiment, organic chemists with their majestic disregard for human variation can pontificate about the reliability of method at low levels.

When it comes to progesterone, the problems are in some ways easier and in others more difficult. Progesterone metabolizes primarily to pregnanediol. However, unfortunately, pregnenolone, pregnenolone sulfate, and 20α and 20β reduced metabolites also come out as pregnanediol. Thus, a measure of pregnanediol includes not only progesterone but also metabolites of these four precursor compounds. Contemporary methods have been greatly simplified over the old ones. We have made a comparison at different levels of output between a silica gel method that we published back in 1962 (which is very specific and extremely laborious) and a much more rapid gas chromatographic method. They are in adequate agreement for clinical purposes.

Interestingly, there is no diurnal variation with pregnanediol and therefore it is not necessary to take a 24-hour urine sample. One can measure pregnanediol on a timed overnight sample, for example, when studying the effectiveness of oral contraceptive compounds.

If these remarks have produced a great feeling of insecurity, you may be certain that the dynamic methods for secretion rates are not going to be the answer to all these problems either.

In theory, the dynamic tests that Dr. Lloyd mentioned are wonderful. One injects an isotope, waits for it to dilute in the body compartment, measures the specific activity of the diluted material, and there you are. Unfortunately, there are a large number of inherent mathematical assumptions involved, and none of them can be taken lightly. And unfortunately, the more we learn about the isotope dilution method with urinary metabolites, the more situations arise where one or more of these basic assumptions is violated and the determination is invalid.

In summary, may I apologize for speaking to you in such a destructive fashion. You may discount much of what I say; I hope, however, that I have left you with a healthy distrust of the figures provided by clinical endocrine laboratories and that this will give you increased reliance on clinical criteria when it comes to the evaluation of androgenic, estrogenic, or progestational effects.

4

Metropathia Hemorrhagica and Nonpsychogenic Amenorrhea

Anna L. Southam, M.D.

It's very hard to know what to say in response to such an introduction, so I just want to say good morning ladies and gentlemen, it's a pleasure to be here. I'd like to expand my title and talk about all the symptoms of menstrual abnormalities that we find in adolescents or in adults. They are the same; they have the same significance. Oligomenorrhea, primary and secondary amenorrhea, and metropathia hemorrhagica or dysfunctional bleeding are deviations from a normal or average menstrual pattern. They are nonspecific symptoms or signs. They have no diagnostic significance in themselves and, in fact, may have exactly the same etiology. A woman with disturbed ovarian function at one time may have dysfunctional bleeding, but at another time, amenorrhea or oligomenorrhea. So here we are with a group of symptoms that are just about as specific as the symptom of pain or headache. The question is sometimes asked, how do you treat amenorrhea? You don't treat amenorrhea; you investigate it and treat the cause of the menstrual abnormality. Definitions vary a little bit so I'd like first to present the definitions that I'm going to use and talk about differential diagnosis. Oligomenorrhea describes a menstrual pattern in which bleeding occurs at longer than usual intervals. Generally, we consider the interval to be longer than six weeks and less than a year. Oligomenorrhea may be a normal adolescent pattern or it may be a pattern that is established during adolescence and continues for the lifetime of the individual. We use the term oligo-ovulatory because this implies that although menses are infrequent they are always preceded by ovulation. The implications and the prognosis are somewhat different in the group of oligo-ovulators than in the group of oligomenorrheic women or adolescents who are anovulatory. The normal adolescent pattern may be characterized by ovulatory oligomenorrhea. Oligomenorrhea which is anovulatory may alternate with episodes of severe dysfunctional bleeding or with periods of amenorrhea. This pattern may also be characteristic of the normal adolescent menstrual pattern. I think we might consider here for a moment what the normal adolescent pattern is. Dr. Vollman collected 5575 cycles in 216 women from menarche to maturity and evaluated them by the means of the basal body temperature chart, a magnificent accomplishment.[3] Vollman introduced the term gynecological age and designated menarche as gynecological year one since it is his feeling that gynecological age is more important than chronological age. He feels it may take as long as 10 years after menarche for an individual to develop a mature menstrual pattern and that menstrual experience is the most important factor. His definition of adolescence would therefore cover the 10 years following menarche. This might place the end of adolescence at 19 years with early menarche or as late as 27 or 28 years in those individuals who had a late onset of menarche. In his study, he shows that the cycle length and the cycle variability decrease progressively with each year after menarche and finally the average duration approaches the 28-day interval which is considered average or normal. He found that during the first year after menarche 55 per cent of cycles were anovulatory. Only 18 per cent of adolescent cycles were associated with a luteal phase, a postovulatory phase, of 10 days or more. This incidence of lack of ovulation decreased progressively until by the 11th or 12th gynecological year only 2.9 per cent of these individuals remained anovulatory. Lack of ovulation is physiological during adolescence and it is usually associated with a normal bleeding pattern. Few of Dr. Vollman's 216 patients required any particular therapy for prolonged bleeding due to lack of ovulation. Let's define metropathia hemorrhagica. I prefer the term dysfunctional bleeding, but some use the term functional uterine bleeding. It's characterized by profuse and sometimes life threatening hemorrhage. The heavy blood loss usually follows episodes of amenorrhea or oligomenorrhea. It may characterize the very first menstrual period of an adolescent. Differential diagnosis includes exclusion of the complications of pregnancy, exclusion of genital tract lesions, and exclusion of systemic disease, including some of the hemorrhagic systemic diseases. I think I can best illustrate this point by telling you what we found in an adolescent group that was admitted for curettage.[1] Between the years of 1920 and 1958, a 38-year period, there were 500 individuals less than the age of 20 admitted to Sloane Hospital for curettage. The majority of these 500 young women were admitted for some complication of pregnancy or incomplete abortion. Ovarian cysts or corpus luteum cysts were found in a few instances. Organic abnormalities were rare. There were only three or four cases of cervical or endometrial polyps. There was one case of documented hypothyroidism, one of pelvic tuberculosis, and one of idiopathic thrombocytopenia. This left 118 adolescents admitted during a 38-year period who seemed to fit the category of dysfunctional bleeding. I'll go back to this group a little bit later. Besides the hospital series in which followup is incomplete, we have a series in the Sloane Endocrine Clinic. Dysfunctional bleeding may be associated with systemic disease, central nervous system lesions, blood dyscrasias, and psychiatric problems. In the normally anovulatory adolescent systemic disease must be exhaustively excluded as a cause of symptoms. I'd like to present briefly just one case, an old one, that illustrates this point. A woman came at the age of 25 for infertility workup. At the age of 16, she had had repeated episodes of dysfunctional bleeding and finally in desperation the gynecologist had used intracavitary radium, not enough to cause permanent cessation of ovarian function but enough to destroy the uterine cavity. Two weeks after this was done, she developed hematuria and the diagnosis of thrombocytopenic purpura was made. She was cured by splenectomy. At the time we studied her several years later ovarian function was normal but she was not menstruating and was infertile. There are a few other causes, I think, of dysfunctional bleeding that we should mention. One is drug therapy. Very serious hemorrhages may occur from the misuse of endocrine therapy. Dysfunctional bleeding may be a transient adolescent pattern or it may be a pattern that will continue into adult life. It may also be one of the early symptoms of the polycystic ovary syndrome. I'll come back a little later to the prognosis and treatment.

Secondary amenorrhea is defined as cessation of menses sometime after menarche. We classify a patient as amenorrheic if her menstrual flow occurs at intervals of one year or longer. However, we also use this term to describe shorter periods of absent menses if the periods have been regular before because we don't know what the menstrual pattern will be. The causes of amenorrhea in the adolescent are similar to those in the adult and the most frequent cause is pregnancy. We must consider uterine factors also. In our adolescents with secondary amenorrhea, we have found tuberculous endometritis and emdometrial destruction following septic abortion. The cause of the amenorrhea may be intrinsic in the ovary with very early primary ovarian failure which may or may not be genetic. The ovary may contain lesions which affect the menstrual pattern and produce amenorrhea by their effect on the hypothalamic pituitary-axis. These would be functioning ovarian tumors and perhaps we'll put polycystic ovaries into this category. Other factors which prevent either the production or release of pituitary stimulating hormones would include central nervous system lesions, pituitary failure, and systemic disease including endocrine abnormalities of the adrenal or the thyroid glands. Amenorrhea may occur in adolescents associated with planned weight loss which is often rapid weight loss and may result in amenorrhea which is rather prolonged. Amenorrhea may be associated with obesity, but again we don't know whether this is coincidental or whether the obesity is the cause of the symptom. Then, of course, there are the psychogenic amenorrheas. The girl going away to college or the nurse in training may present with amenorrhea. An adolescent with a serious psychosis may present first with a menstrual problem or she may present later while on drug therapy. I think it is here that we might remember that tranquilizers may produce amenorrhea in any age group. The diagnosis of psychogenic amenorrhea worries me quite a bit since I don't know how to make it. Here, again, I'd like to present a brief case history. This 18-year-old patient had had one menstrual period at the age of 14 and no more. She had seen a gynecologist and she had seen a psychiatrist and was told that her amenorrhea was psychogenic. She was treated for several months and years by withdrawal therapy until at the age of 17½ she suddenly went blind. At this time, an investigation was done and a large pituitary adenoma found. I believe strongly in psychogenic amenorrhea but I believe very strongly in a complete workup of the adolescent or of anyone, even if obviously neurotic or even psychotic. We are obliged to rule out coexisting disease. The mere fact that a woman does not have menstrual periods may produce a psychological reaction that is secondary rather than the primary cause of her disease. I think the diagnosis of psychogenic amenorrhea is difficult to make and one that can be made only after a great deal of investigation. In a number of cases the diagnosis may not be apparent at the time of the study, *i.e.*, "amenorrhea of unknown etiology." These we follow, and restudy. Occasionally, as we restudy them over the years, organic pathology appears. I do not think the process of investigation stops after the first workup has failed to reveal a cause. If the problem persists, review of the possible causes is indicated in a year or two. Primary amenorrhea simply means that the menses have never occurred. A problem may occur here in history taking. Individuals fail to distinguish between an induced menstrual period and a spontaneous menstrual period, and when we go into details at the history taking, we may find that the individual has had only induced menstrual periods— withdrawal bleeding—and that she has never had a spontaneous period. Women may fail to recognize other sites of blood loss and insist that menstrual periods have occurred even though on examination the vagina or uterus is absent. In primary amenorrhea, there are certain conditions that we don't encounter in secondary amenorrhea. Often the pediatrician has made the diagnosis long before the age of menarche or even shortly after birth. This is true in some patients with gonadal dysgenesis and with congenital adrenal hyperplasia. In primary amenorrhea it is necessary to consider the differential diagnosis of delayed menarche. Sometimes this differential can be made only in retrospect because factors which caused delayed menarche may be exactly the same as those that cause primary amenorrhea or secondary amenorrhea. It may be only after a period of observation that this diagnosis can be made; patients with delayed menarche are entitled to the same type of investigation as the patients with primary amenorrhea or secondary amenorrhea. If we exclude the congenital and genetic anomalies, primary amenorrhea has the same causes as secondary amenorrhea. Our collection of girls with primary amenorrhea includes individuals who have pelvic tuberculosis; one had her first menstrual period at the age of 26 after antituberculous therapy. It includes patients with central nervous system lesions and pituitary tumors, patients with ovarian tumors, and patients with polycystic ovaries. Systemic diseases associated with primary amenorrhea include cases of portal hypertension, hypoparathyroidism, thyrotoxicosis, hypothyroidism, severe juvenile diabetes, and hemolytic anemia. Of course, nutritional factors are important here too. We consider exactly the same things that we do in secondary amenorrhea after we have ruled out the congenital and genetic abnormalities.

These are definitions and possible causes. Somehow we have to find out what the symptoms mean. We might have to do it without the aid of a laboratory since Dr. Goldzieher tells us that laboratory tests may not give the answer. A great deal can be learned about the patient without laboratory examinations and without the help of the endocrine laboratory, although I believe it is very important and very helpful. History is one of the important diagnostic methods and includes a complete history—the age at which various secondary sex characteristics appeared and the time of onset of the menstrual abnormality. We inquire about the mother's menstrual history, the grandmother's, the aunts' and the siblings'. I don't know what this tells us, but the mother likes to tell it. A complete system review must be done. Somewhere in the process of taking a history and doing a system review, we explain to the girl, and to the mother if she's there, the basic steps involved in menstruation. She often knows this but we review them so that she knows what we're going to be looking for and why we need certain tests. A complete physical examination follows and this along with the history gives clues to guide the laboratory investigation. We do, in almost all instances, either a rectal or vaginal examination or both unless there are cultural objections to this, and if we can do them without pain. We might remember that some of the patients with dysfunctional bleeding have had previous examinations under anesthesia and previous curettages. We can do a pelvic or a rectovaginal examination without hurting them. Remember that many girls these days use tampax, at least part of the time. If an adolescent is using tampax, there is no reason why one cannot do a gentle one-finger pelvic examination. Girls these days are taught something about menstrual function and reproductive physiology in the 7th and 8th grade and they're taught this in their hygiene courses in high school. The girl that comes with a menstrual abnormality is concerned. She knows that menstrual function is tied up with reproductive physiology, and she's going to wonder how you can know if there's anything wrong with her uterus or her ovaries if you don't examine that system as well as her heart and lungs and her breasts. The reproductive organs are as important as any other system in the body, and as easy, usually, to examine as any other system. I think that if the physician approaches this in a matter-of-fact way, the adolescent will feel no sense of shame or no sense of reluctance about this type of examination. After the routine physical examination, I merely say to the patient that I will examine her uterus and ovaries. I explain to her what a bimanual examination is, and that she must relax. Most do this very well. I want to stress again that there are cultural and religious contra-indications to doing this, and then we never do it. When this examination is finished, and the girl is told that everything is normal her face lights up. I also think that a girl with a menstrual abnormality should have her own gynecologist, not her mother's gynecologist, and that she should feel that the gynecologist is her own and is not a parent but a friend and a counselor and a physician that she can talk to about anything.

Laboratory tests should be ordered as needed. We usually do blood counts, urinalyses, and chest x-rays if the child has never had one. The indicated endocrine function tests are done. Abnormal findings rarely come as a complete surprise after history and physical examination.

It is important to determine the degree of ovarian function or ovarian failure. Sometimes inspection of the external genitalia and the introitus will reveal atrophy which suggests that there is very little estrogen effect. Vaginal smears can be taken in most adolescents and are useful. We can evaluate cytology also from urinary sediment. If it is possible to insert a small speculum into the vagina, cervical mucus and vaginal epithelium can be evaluated. The appearance of cervical mucus is a very valuable index of estrogen production. It is useful to administer a single injection of 50 mg. of progesterone. If there is enough endogenous estrogen being produced to cause a proliferative endometrium, withdrawal bleeding will occur. If withdrawal bleeding occurs after injection of progesterone only, the individual has some endometrial development. Gonadotropins will not be elevated, there is a lack of ovulation, but some estrogen is being produced. If no bleeding follows progesterone administration, it becomes necessary to distinguish between estrogen lack due to primary ovarian failure, and estrogen lack due to absence of stimulation from the central nervous system. In this situation, gonadotropin assays are very useful, and unequivocally elevated values indicate primary ovarian failure. I would find it quite difficult to get along without gonadotropin assays in this group of individuals. It may be that, as exogenous gonadotropins become more generally available, we can use these as a diagnostic test. End organ failure must be ruled out. Here we could expect normal ovarian function but absent withdrawal bleeding from both progesterone and from estrogen. Very often the adolescent will be interested in taking six or eight weeks of basal body temperature, and this is one way of proving uterine failure; serial pregnanediols could be done but a basal body temperature chart is cheaper and easier. If withdrawal bleeding occurs from estrogen, the endometrium is capable of responding to the appropriate hormones and this finding essentially rules out uterine amenorrhea. In the group with no withdrawal bleeding from progesterone and with low gonadotropins, an x-ray of the sella is very important. If the x-ray of the sella is normal, visual fields examination may be indicated. We have restudied individuals and picked up pituitary tumors later that were not apparent on previous examinations.

I'd like to consider the prognosis for adolescents with various menstrual abnormalities. Very often, women date the onset of a menstrual abnormality to the adolescent years, but only women with certain abnormalities. In general, women with amenorrhea due to organic pathology do not give a history of adolescent menstrual irregularity or abnormalities that were significant enough for them to remember. Hence 86 per cent of a group of 127 gave a history of a normal adolescent menstrual pattern. In patients with menstrual dysfunction of undetermined etiology, we have the reverse. This group includes many patients who later fell into the category of Stein-Leventhal syndrome; 78 per cent had an abnormal adolescent menstrual pattern. Four patients developed endometrial carcinoma before the end of the usual reproductive life. Patients with polycystic ovaries most usually date the onset of menstrual abnormalities to adolescent years; often there is a curettage during adolescence; often they remember prolonged treatment for menstrual abnormalities. In our series 93 per cent had abnormal menses since before the age of 20. The adolescent menstrual histories of some women were sent to the endocrine clinic with the diagnosis of dysfunctional bleeding; it was found that benign uterine pathology was the cause of the abnormal bleeding. Again, the majority of patients remembered no significant abnormality during adolescence. The adolescent menstrual history of patients seen for postpartum difficulties, persistent postpartum bleeding which was not thought to be due to the pregnancy, with oligomenorrhea or with amenorrhea indicated that the majority of women remembered no abnormality during their adolescence. Perhaps the retrospective history is of some value. I might comment here on the value of the retrospective history of menarche too. It was pointed out yesterday that this is one of the most important events that occur in the life of an individual, and that the next most important event is the birth of a child. A mother doesn't forget the birthday of her child and very often a woman can give you the day and the month and the year and what happened on that day of her first menstrual period. She might not remember when her last menstrual period was or the period before, but she remembers her first period.

   Let's go now to some smaller studies that we have in progress that are prospective studies. When we study the adults we get a concentration of abnormal women, and this does not give an indication of what the risk is for the adolescent with a menstrual abnormality.[2] These are adolescents seen for various menstrual abnormalities of undetermined etiology. There is no point in including the organic cases here because those should be treated and not followed. The numbers are small because it takes time to follow an adolescent for 10 years postmenarche, and some of our cases we lose. In 13 patients who had amenorrhea of undetermined etiology during adolescence, 9 remained abnormal for more than 10 years after menarche. Of 32 patients with oligomenorrhea, only 4 established the conventional cycle of 28 days, plus or minus a few days, and 28 continued to be oligomenorrheic. Of 58 patients with dysfunctional bleeding, 17 were normal 10 years after menarche while 41 continued to have a menstrual abnormality, either amenorrhea or oligomenorrhea associated with abnormal bleeding. Now what about the subsequent fertility of these particular patients? We'll consider first the patients with amenorrhea. In the group that reverted to normal within the 10 years after menarche, we know of 9 marriages and 8 have proven fertility. If the menstrual pattern becomes normal, it has no effect on subsequent reproductive function. In the patients with secondary amenorrhea who remained abnormal, 5 were married and only 1 had a pregnancy. This is not persistent amenorrhea; this is any menstrual pattern in which there is bleeding at more than a one-year interval; these people occasionally ovulate and menstruate. We have one patient that was amenorrheic from the age of 20 to the age of 43 when she had her first child. The oligomenorrheic patients are rather interesting. Although this pattern persisted into adulthood, these women were not particularly infertile. In this group of 28 that maintained their oligomenorrheic pattern, we know that 15 are married and 10 are pregnant. I am sure that as our duration of follow-up increases pregnancies will also increase. So oligo-ovulation may simply be a variation from the average pattern. Oligomenorrhea if it is ovulatory, does not have a particularly bad prognosis.

In patients with dysfunctional bleeding, in the group of 41 that remained abnormal, 14 were married and no pregnancies had occurred at the time these statistics were put together. Go back for a minute to the series of 118 patients admitted for curettage during adolescence; 41 of these patients, a third, required more than one curettage.[1] Remember, many of these were in the days before progestin therapy, and I present them just to show what the natural history might be. Some of these had as many as 8 curettages with anesthesia, with blood transfusions, and so forth. Eight patients in the group of 41 requiring repeated curettages had hysterectomies quite early in their reproductive life and 3 hysterectomies were performed before the patients were 10 years postmenarche. Eighteen in this group have been followed for 11 to 36 years after menarche and there are 2 cases of endometrial carcinoma. The prognosis associated with untreated dysfunctional bleeding can be quite serious.

I wanted to illustrate the fact that menstrual patterns vary in a single individual. I think I might do this with a couple of case histories. One individual presented with primary amenorrhea at the age of 18. At that time, she simply had a proliferative endometrium. At age 21, without any normal menstrual periods, she developed a pattern of abnormal bleeding. Curettage at that time again showed a proliferative endometrium. She had repeated episodes of pelvic inflammatory disease but her anovulatory pattern continued. Her endometrium at the age of 30 is a proliferative type of endometrium, not particularly worrisome, perhaps with a little nuclear crowding. The endometrium of the next patient, an 18-year-old girl with dysfunctional bleeding, showed a mildly cystic pattern and that's all. At the age of 27, she had another curettage which showed again some cystic hyperplasia and that's about all. At the time of her wedge resection, we found a little more glandular hyperplasia, perhaps a little minimal budding into some of the glandular lumina but not a particularly bad endometrium. This woman, with a lifelong history of menstrual abnormality, responded well to wedge resection with normal ovulatory cycles at the age of 34. The next patient was a woman who had had menstrual abnormalities since shortly after menarche. She was 28 when a sample of endometrium was taken. It showed a considerable amount of atypical hyperplasia, enough to worry some of the pathologists, and again this was a woman with a problem, since menarche, of amenorrhea and abnormal bleeding. At the time of this study she had had a year of amenorrhea. A wedge resection was done. She has had 3 children since and her endometrium is normal. We follow all of our adolescent patients with past menstrual abnormalities if we can, because we find a recurrent pattern particularly with dysfunctional bleeding. The fact that a woman has a baby may not mean that she's going to continue to have normal menstrual function and normal reproductive function. Two weeks ago we restudied a girl seen previously for adolescent bleeding. She had had 2 children and came with a year of amenorrhea. Biopsy showed adenocarcinoma of the endometrium. The next patient is a 30-year-old woman presenting with primary amenorrhea. Her endometrial biopsy showed an endometrial adeno-acanthoma. I present these cases just to emphasize the fact that adolescent menstrual abnormalities are important. They may be the onset of a really serious disease.

Adolescents with dysfunctional bleeding are treated to produce cyclic withdrawal bleeding. We use progesterone 50 mg. intramuscularly every five weeks or so. This will give the patient a chance to have a normal menstrual period if she ovulates before she receives the drug. If she doesn't bleed in the expected time after the injection of progesterone, it probably means that she has ovulated. Usually withdrawal bleeding in the anovulatory individuals occurs in 4½ to 5 days after injection of progesterone. We also treat some of our amenorrheic patients with cyclic withdrawal bleeding from progesterone, again a single injection on a single day. These are the patients that have endogenous estrogens and many of them are happier if they have an occasional period. We don't necessarily treat them in cyclic fashion as we do with dysfunctional bleeding. Patients with lack of endogenous estrogen need replacement therapy, at least for a period of time to develop secondary sex characteristics. Some of the adolescents that have a persistent abnormality will turn out to have Stein-Leventhal syndrome when we study them later. They respond to wedge resection. In our series the response to wedge resection is just as good at the age of 28 or even 38 as it is at 18, and I would prefer to treat these young patients symptomatically to see if they establish a normal menstrual pattern before we do surgical procedures. There is some indication that the normal adolescent ovary may have a polycystic pattern; there may be many expanded follicles, absent corpora lutea. In fact, some of the histological sections that we have obtained from autopsies on adolescent girls appear very similar, indeed, to the Stein-Leventhal ovary. The pathologist will make a diagnosis of an ovary consistent with Stein-Leventhal syndrome although the patient really had none of the symptoms that go with it. Ovulation can be induced with gonadotropins. I don't think these have much of a place in the routine management of the adolescent girl. They might be used for diagnosis. In general the ovulation inducing drugs and definitive measures for inducing ovulation might well wait until the individual is a little more mature. Wedge resections might be indicated during late adolescence and considered as more conservative than admitting the patient for repeated curettages and repeated blood transfusions if she fails to come back for substitution therapy.

In closing, I'd like to say that the patient with amenorrhea may present first to the gynecologist or to the pediatrician and it is his responsibility to see that this individual is completely worked up. The physician may not be able to complete the work-up himself but this is where the patient comes first as she deserves more than just pills. The psychiatrist, the psychologist, the neurologist, the neurosurgeon, the internist, the endocrinologist, the biochemist, the geneticist, the surgeon, the radiotherapist all have a part in either the diagnosis or in the treatment of menstrual abnormalities.

REFERENCES

1. Southam, A. L.: Dysfunctional uterine bleeding in adolescence. Clinical Obst. & Gynec., *3:* 241, 1960.
2. Southam, A. L.: The natural history of menstrual disorders. Ann. New York Acad. Sci., *75:* 840, 1959.
3. Vollman, R. F.: Patterns of menstrual performance in adolescent girls. Proc. 2nd World Congress on Fertil. & Steril., Naples, p. 27, 1956.

5

The Management of Congenital Defects

Somers H. Sturgis, M.D.

It is perfectly obvious, of course, from what we have heard this morning from Dr. Southam and from Dr. Marbach and the panelists yesterday that any dysfunction of the adolescent reproductive system is loaded with emotional connotations. We can appreciate the confusion which is added to the chaos of adolescence if there is some anatomical deviation in the genital system. Defects in genital anatomy may need hormonal or surgical correction—but, obviously, they cannot escape having to be dealt with on an emotional level as well, because of the huge investment of the young person in the question, "who am I, am I a boy or am I a girl?" I think it is appropriate to review first some of the chief causes of congenital defects in adolescents and speak of their diagnosis before we get to their management. Mankind has always been intrigued with the whole subject of intersex. Back in the third century B.C. we find mentions of the union of Hermes and Aphrodite and the formation of an individual that had elements of both sexes. Ovid, I believe, embellished this somewhat in one of his tales in the first century describing a beautiful Apollo, a 15-year-old boy who goes narcissistically to look at his image in a pool. A naiad springs from the pool, falls desperately in love with him, and drags him down with her into the water, praying to the gods that they will never be separated. Her prayers are answered and they become fused into one person, Hermaphrodites, or the first hermaphrodite, so says the poet. The curiosity certainly intrigued the artists, the sculptors, and so on, of the early centuries. Examples are readily found in the frescoes of Pompeii. These characters were godlike, they were worshipped, they were thought to be more than human and they were to be taken care of. We have the same morbid curiosity about cases like that of Christine Jorgenson. Bradbury has reported a case of an individual who was born and operated on at 6 years of age with the testis on one side and an ovary on the other. Indeed, there are laboratory experiments of intrauterine embryonic trauma that have produced a half male and half female animal.

The pediatrician or the obstetrician is faced with a real problem when a baby is born with ambiguous external paraphernalia. He must decide then and there the sex of the child. I couldn't agree more with what Dr. Gardiner said yesterday about the importance of his decision. The young mother who, perhaps, had "natural" childbirth looks up expectantly and says, "Well, what is it doctor?" And he says, "I don't know, I've got to look at the inside of the mouth." Her reaction may be, "Well, what kind of a doctor are you that you don't know where to look?" There can be every kind and variety of ambiguity, of course, with normal external genitalia but defective internal organs or *vice versa,* and all types of varieties between the two. Doctor Gardiner said yesterday, "it isn't the chromosomes, it isn't the hormones that are important to this child, it's the decision made at birth as to the sex of rearing."

The genetic sex is that which establishes the gonadal sex and this in turn gives rise to the body sex which has three facets. First are the internal structures; second are the external genitalia, which are going to give the orientation of sexuality to the newborn child. This will also decide how he is going to consider himself, and deal with other individuals, setting the pattern of social behavior that is going to be with him all his life. The third factor is the gonadal hormone secretions. If we have a genetic male brought up as a female into adolescence and beginning to mature, this individual can be changed perfectly well by plastic surgery into a female type that she was reared to be. This isn't difficult at all. But if you have a genetic female brought up as a male, it's impossible, of course, to create a functional phallus that will be any good in marital relations. If there is any question and the laboratory is not there to help one decide, the preference should be to call this ambiguous child a female because this can be supported with hormones and with plastic surgery, so this individual can be helped to lead a perfectly normal, functional, marital life. Laboratory tests are certainly helpful. The buccal smear will show the Barr body, a chromatin body on the edge of the nuclear membrane of buccal epithelial cells. In a recent study of 50 normal males and 50 normal females at our hospital we got up to 4 per cent positive chromatin Barr bodies in the normal males. We never had less than 10 per cent in our female population. Interesting enough, similar results were found in a study done at Yale. Generally, no matter what techniques a laboratory uses, there will be no overlapping. Most laboratories nowadays find no Barr bodies; if they find one or two in a normal male, they consider them artifacts. This is an easy test to do. I am surprised that obstetrical services do not require that this be done in all newborns. It would seem to me such a simple and nontraumatic way to pick up numbers of cases that would not be discovered for some years later. However, it isn't infallible because "mosaics" may be misleading as far as the single buccal smear test goes. There are also "drumsticks" in the neutrophils of the peripheral blood smear in the female, which, as you recall, are not found in the genetic male, and the female may have up to 4 per cent or so.

Then, of course, there is the "squash" technique of the *in vitro* incubation of epithelial cells which gives the karyotype when the chromosomes are arrested in metaphase. These can be put on a piece of paper according to the Denver classification. I certainly cannot tell you why one chromosome is an X and another isn't an X but the geneticists know and can make such differentiations. This is such a highly specialized field that it is almost impossible for any of us to feel that we can be any more than amateurs in this line now, and we have to rely on the laboratory to help us determine the karyotype. We should review briefly some of the anatomical defects that give abnormal genetic patterns. Attention should be focused on the importance of the Y chromosome which causes gonadal differentiation to the male sex whenever it occurs. It does not matter how many X's you have, that Y is the one that causes the development of testes and male external genitalia. Only one of the two X's in the normal female gives the Barr body, so the formula for the number of Barr bodies is X minus 1. If you have two or three Barr bodies the number will be one less than the number of X's in your genetic constitution. If something goes wrong in division of the germ cell in meiosis, one can get defects by nondisjunction, a failure of the proper division of the chromosomes. This would then give rise to an X-O individual or an XXY. But nondisjunction can occur after the original reduction and division of the germ cell. It can occur in mitosis in embryonic life, and this individual then is a mosaic. The mosaicisms that are being reported nowadays are infinite and intriguing.

The term hermaphrodite, whether it's male or female, of course, relates to the gonadal sex of the individual. The true hermaphrodite is an individual with both testes and ovaries or elements of testes and ovary present. These are not very common. Actually, I have only taken care of one. This condition may either be present at birth or it may be acquired. The case in my experience was that of a 15-year-old girl who had the menarche at 13 and menstruated quite normally for a year. Then her periods stopped. During the last year she began to grow hair on her face, her voice became husky, and her clitoris was enlarged; but her breast development was excellent and vaginal smear showed good cornification. We did not really know what we were getting into. The 17-ketosteroids were normal and urinary gonadotropins were in normal range. She was explored and we found a tumor in one ovary. Histologically this tumor had features that were thought to be testicular with an occasional tubular structure. In addition, there were elements interpreted to be granulosa cells. This was a gynandroblastoma, producing both androgenic and estrogenic hormones. Removal of the ovary with the tumor, happily, did reverse her hirsutism. Maybe Dr. Greenblatt will comment on the reversibility or irreversibility of hirsutism in his cases. In this girl periods came back, her voice didn't change, but her superfluous hair did go away, and she was very pleased.

The female pseudohermaphrodite, a confusing term, means someone who has ovaries, whose genotype is female, but in whom there are evidences of ambiguity in the external genitalia. This is typical of congenital adrenal hyperplasia. It has occurred in daughters of mothers who were given certain hormones in the first trimester which proved androgenic so the female child was born with an enlarged clitoris, or phallus. Such a female pseudo-hermaphrodite can be taken care of surgically with a clitorectomy. Most congenital adrenal hyperplasia patients have perfectly good Müllerian structures, the uterus and vagina. They may have a common urogenital sinus and need a plastic surgical repair to open up the introitus and vestibule. They can be helped tremendously by proper surgery. After all, our major aim is to try to conform to the genotype as best we can and to try to help this individual to be as normal in function as her anatomy will allow.

The male pseudohermaphrodite challenges us with a different kind of situation. I'd like to illustrate this by the case of an individual with the testicular feminization syndrome, in which the clinical diagnosis is made easily by a simple physical examination. This was a 17-year-old girl who came into the office last summer. She was very well developed, better endowed than many of her classmates in terms of mammary development. She had no pubic or axillary hair at all; this is the pathognomic feature. It is not necessary to go any further after finding this discrepancy—lack of axillary or public hair—in a well developed, very feminine girl. Diagnosis, of course, can be confirmed by the chromosomal analysis which will be XY, and a buccal smear which will be negative. Her history was very suggestive and helpful, in that she was said by the mother to have had a "hernia" operation in one groin when she was a year old. Suspecting the diagnosis from the physical examination, I palpated the other groin very carefully, and said, "Yes, I'm afraid you've got a hernia on the other side, too. It must be fixed." She said, "I'm getting married this winter, so let's get it done." This gave me the chance to do an orchiectomy on the other side. These conditions may run in families. Her sister was 15 and had exactly the same thing. The important thing in management is to do everything possible to prevent any leak of the diagnosis to get to the girl or her family. If my patient ever had heard something mentioned about a testis when she was in the hospital I believe it would have destroyed her whole life. When she came into the hospital, her record was locked up in the nurse's desk, because students or student nurses may hear about an interesting case, about a girl who may be a boy, and run to the record and pore over it. It is important to alert everybody who has anything to do with the case not to take it casually. The attitude must be maintained that this is merely a youngster who has a hernia; she is going to have it fixed; she had a lump when she was born and she has a lump on the other side that's going to be fixed now. If one can keep any suggestion of the diagnosis from such a young lady, it is best for her. If, on the other hand, it leaks out in some way or other, irreparable harm may be done. She will be in a chaotic emotional confusion; her impending marriage and probably any future marriage ideas will be wrecked. As you have gathered, I feel very strongly that the gonads should be removed in these cases. The oponents of this view say, but isn't this the only source of hormones that she has? Isn't this giving her a good female figure? Aren't you castrating her? How can you do this? Nevertheless, I think there are two very strong reasons for doing the orchiectomy. There are several reports that as high as 40 per cent of these unusual abnormal testes will degenerate in later life into malignancy. Then the first reason for removing them is the possibility of malignant degeneration and this goes hand in hand with a second, in my opinion, more powerful reason. Since malignancy is a possibility, it is the doctor's responsibility to have the girl come in once every 6 months or so and carefully palpate the groin, for any change in the undescended gonad. As the months and years go by, I would think it would be almost impossible for this individual not to finally say, but, doctor, why are you so interested? Why do you have to do this? For heaven's sake, what's wrong? The doctor's job is to explain the hormonal deficiency to his patient. Some people are born, for instance, with poor thyroids and have to have thyroid all their lives; some people are born with a not very good pancreas, are diabetics, and have to take insulin. In this case, the ovaries just didn't develop very well, and therefore there is the need to take hormones indefinitely. Since these individuals are castrated, they do need estrogen. They obviously don't have any Müllerian system so they don't have any uterus. The girl has a perfectly good vagina but no tubes and no uterus. Stilbestrol, 1 mg., may be given daily without worrying about bleeding or it can be interrupted with progesterone pills, like Pranone, 10 mg., four times a day for three or four days each month. This is said to give the cyclicity that some people say is best for maintenance of breasts. I don't know whether it is important or not.

The most common of the genetic defects in the adolescent female certainly would be the Turner's group. We have had 35 cases of Turner's syndrome diagnosed in the last 15 years or so at Dr. Gallagher's Adolescent Clinic. There have been many more in the Children's Hopsital. These adolescents have a height of not more than 54 in., and, as Dr. Albright mentioned back in 1936, together with short stature, genital infantilism, and amenorrhea, one has to document a high total gonadotropin output. In the clinic or in the office it is not always easy to make the diagnosis. There are three definite ways of making the diagnosis. Either it is necessary to have a karyotype which shows mosaicism or a 45 XO configuration, a laparotomy with the demonstration of the streak ovaries, or elevated follicle stimulating hormone (FSH). Dr. Southam brought out this morning that one will be fooled by some late maturers. In our 35 cases admitted with a tentative diagnosis of Turner's syndrome, there were six that did not have a high FSH and we held our diagnosis and waited. Two of these were operated on and turned out to have gonadal dysgenesis. The other four eventually came around at 17 or 18, with a little bit of pubic hair and mammary development starting and eventually came to the menarche at over 18. One must be sure of his diagnosis, and in our clinic we insist on an elevated FSH. But how elevated must it be? We feel that if the patient has an FSH test positive for 50 mouse units and yet has genital infantilism and no evidence of estrogen, then a diagnosis of Turner's syndrome certainly can be made. It is not necessary to have 100 or 200 or 300 units. The karyotype may be misleading if one has mosaics, and the typical features that we read about in textbooks are also misleading. In our cases, as in the literature, about 80 per cent were "XO," but there were mosaics that were chromatin positive. Many of the 17 ketosteroid excretions were low, about the level of a 5- or 6-year-old child. Some of the girls that were taller had a more normal ketosteroid output, suggesting that the adrenals may have something to do with increased height. There are other features that are of some interest. The urinary cytology can be helpful in adolescents as an appraisal of their estrogen output.

Dr. McArthur spoke of this and showed some pictures in the first lecture yesterday, and Dr. Southam mentioned it again today. In a young adolescent, particularly in one with Turner's syndrome who looks about 6 or 8 years old (although her age is 14 or 15) and is afraid of anything that may happen, a vaginal smear probably is not justified. However, a first voided urine specimen is simple to collect and can be added to one-third its volume of alcohol, spun down, and smeared as with a Papanicolaou smear. The cells washed down as sediment from the lower urethra permit a very good assay for estrogen production. A few years ago Dr. Castellanos, working in our laboratory, was very much interested in urinary cytology. He first noted the presence of degenerated cells that are nonnucleated and appear in any situation where there is an absence of ovarian estrogen. These nonnucleated cells may make up a large per cent of the cellular components of a urinary smear in these cases but they don't appear in the vaginal smear. The finding in a voided specimen of a high per cent of nonnucleated cells is a helpful confirmatory diagnostic aid in ovarian dysgenesis. Dr. Castellanos never found more than 20 per cent of nonnucleated cells in a normal individual. Anything over this was abnormal. In the polycystic ovary group more non-nucleated cells are found, and in some of the adolescents that we are studying for developing polycystic ovaries, we look for a high per cent of nonnucleated cells even before the full blown syndrome is readily diagnosed. What happens to these nonnucleated cells if estrogen is given? With adequate estrogen there is a rapid reversal. Obviously, these cells are a reflection of a poorly developed intermediate cell layer from the lower urethra that is not covered with squamous epithelium and these intermediate cells degenerate fast; they appear as just "junk" that most cytologists don't pay attention to. The keratinized degenerated bits can be easily picked out by someone who is familiar with this technique. Urinary cytology can be very helpful in some of these diagnostic problems.

Having made the diagnosis, how about treatment? When are we going to start? We know that the absence of estrogen is associated with osteoporosis in these youngsters; indeed, by the early 20's some of them begin to show osteoporosis if they have not had any estrogens. They need estrogen to protect their bones and also their blood vessels. Psychological and psychiatric studies have been done on a small group of these youngsters in our clinic resulting in some interesting findings. They seem to have a denial of their own body structure. Many of them refuse to recognize that they are different from their peers. Of course, they're different; they "know" they're different. They're "little" people and the rest of their classmates are tall, but they will not accept this; they will often not look at their height realistically. This can be shown quite nicely in a simple psychological test. Give these children a pencil and a piece of paper and say "draw a person." One of them broke down completely. She couldn't do it, refused. Another girl had difficulty in drawing a person, in creating her body image. Her mother told us that she wouldn't have a mirror in her room, that if she tried to put a mirror in her room the daughter would break it. She just would not look at herself. So the physician is confronted with tremendous denial of the youngster's own body image. We feel an effort should be made to try to help them into psychological acceptance of their difficulty before starting them off with Stilbestrol to develop their breasts and give them menstrual periods. In an earlier experience we had one or two patients who would not cooperate at all. They would be given Stilbestrol; they wouldn't take it; they called on every subterfuge not to take their dose. Menstrual flow was to some of these disagreeable, nasty; they didn't want to be grown up. This is just a warning that it is necessary, if possible, to give such patients psychological aid to prepare them for "menarche" or nothing will be gained in treatment. We generally give them Stilbestrol, 1 mg. a day, for the first 3 weeks of each month, and that will give them some sort of withdrawal flow. Maybe some of them need 2 mg. a day. One is not treating hot flashes because they don't have hot flashes. One is not primarily treating the nonunion of epiphyses. Unfortunately, the thing that they want most is to grow, and it is known that with Stilbestrol it will take a ½ or 2 years for the epiphyses to fuse and one to two inches will be gained but that is all that will result. It is best to try to develop the thesis that the pills are going to make them grown-up girls like their classmates. They will get some growth but they must realize how nice it is to be "petite." One of the things I just want to mention is the sexuality of these youngsters. They have been neuters all their life, with neither male nor female hormones, and some have been very tomboyish. What is going to happen to their sexuality when we start to give them female hormones? I remember one that came in blue jeans; her mother was out working all day, paying no attention to this youngster, but she was very close to her father. She had a couple of brothers and she loved to play sports with them. We used to have a game in which we would try to guess whether these little people were going to be mosaics with XO-XX chromosomes, or whether they're going to be plain XO's. We thought this little girl was going to be an XO, but she turned out to be a mosaic with an XX-XO configuration. Some of them are like this. Would they change? Would they begin to put on lipstick and dresses when we gave them estrogen? This girl didn't turn out to be that way. Similarly, when we guessed that the little doll-like girl with the frilly dress would surely be an XX-XO mosaic, she happened to be the XO. In all cases, it isn't the hormone that changes them in their orientation and makes them little girls interested in boys and dating at all. It depends on the mature adult figure that they have identified with, whether it is a father in one case and they're little tomboys, or whether it's a warm, feminine mother or mother figure in the other case where they are "little girls." Some of them don't even respond to Stilbestrol. One had a double uterus and I imagine there is a fairly high incidence of Mullerian anomalies and genitourinary anomalies in this group that one must rightly consider.

I think we must remember that in any young person in whom there is need for surgical reconstruction the time to do it is before the age of 1 or certainly before 2. If this chance has been lost, one must wait until the child is old enough to cooperate, to intelligently understand and accept an explanation of things. This is illustrated by the case of a 17-year-old girl with primary amenorrhea. She had beautiful development, had been the president of her class, and everybody loved her. She had been under the treatment of an endocrinologist in another city. He gave her some shots of Estradiol in good quantities over three months and nothing happened, no menses at all. This is where he missed the boat because he sent her to a surgeon to find out what was wrong. He didn't realize the importance of the absence of any swelling or any suprapubic pain that would be expected if a congenital vaginal atresia or atresia of the cervix was the problem. Given this amount of estrogen, she should have had a hematocolpos develop. She should have had some symptoms from this. She didn't have anything of this sort. The surgeon examined her under anesthesia and found that she had an absent uterus and vagina. He developed a plane of cleavage between the urethra and the rectum and stuffed this full of gauze as an artificial vaginal canal. When this child, who was 17 years old, woke up and was told that she had no reproductive structures and that she needed to keep this gauze replaced and come back and have it repacked every few days, she was completely horrified. She was desperately thwarted in all her hopes of being a normal girl, and she became a recluse. Her studies got so bad she dropped out of school. She would not see her friends; she would not see anybody. She was in miserable condition. Then her mother brought her up to us and asked what should be done. Obviously, she had not cooperated with her surgeon, and the tract that had been formed closed immediately. She did, luckily, have a chance to get a year and a half of psychological help in another city. She came back having reoriented her thoughts and wanting to be fixed. At that time, it was possible to create an artificial vagina with a lining of split graft of skin from the thigh and to give her an obturator which she faithfully used. She got married about a year and a half later and has been married now for four years, apparently normally happy, with normal orgasm and normal vaginal tract. This is to illustrate that you must wait; there is no sense in not getting cooperation from the adolescent if you are going to do something to make her more sexually functional. Hormones and surgery are then helpful aids in supporting the emotional status of the adolescent conditioned almost wholly by the sex of rearing and it is futile to hope that such measures will establish personality structures without a great deal of help in emotional guidance.

6

Ovarian Tumors During Adolescence

Felix P. Heald, M.D.

A pediatrician discussing ovarian tumors as part of such a distinguished faculty is like carrying coals to Newcastle. So, it is with some trepidation that I mount the rostrum today, but there may be some advantage in having an outsider in this particular field discussing ovarian tumors in adolescent girls. The advantage, I think, is particularly to the pediatricians in the audience who know how a pediatrician feels when first confronted with the problem of ovarian tumors. And I will have to make the assumption that the other pediatricians in this room feel as I did in preparing this material. The question can logically be asked, are ovarian tumors in the adolescent girl any different than those in children or adult women? This is a question that Dr. Gallagher, Dr. Sturgis, and I posed to each other a number of years ago, and as a result of this we undertook a study in the Boston area.[2] Over a period of 10 years, from January 1948 to December 1957, all the records on ovarian tumors were gathered from four hospitals. The surgical material came from two general hospitals, the Massachusetts General Hospital and the Peter Bent Brigham Hospital, and, in addition, from the Children's Medical Center in Boston and the Free Hospital for Women. The chronological age of 12 to 21 years was arbitrarily selected for this study group. The fallacy of choosing such an arbitrary chronological age was discussed earlier in the conference. Clinical histories were summarized and made available for correlative purposes. Slides for all the cases reported in this series were reviewed by one of us, Dr. John H. Craig, who recorded a single diagnosis for each tumor. Dr. Ming painstakingly dug through all the records in locating and recording all the clinical data. No limitations were placed on the size of the solid tumors so that some of them were quite small. Ovarian cysts were included in this study if they measured 5 cm. or more. Follicular cysts, cystic corpus luteum, and hemorrhagic corpus luteum were included only if they measured 5 cm. or more. Endometriosis of the ovary was included only when the ovary was 3 times normal size. It should be noted that most of the teratomas in our classification were called dermoids. In those tumors in which only skin elements were included, the term teratoma dermoid was used. The results of this study were then tabulated and we will present them now.

In the 10-year period, there were 72 tumors in 71 girls. In one girl, there was a simple cyst of the ovary as well as a cystadenofibroma. The distribution of the tumors among the four hospitals can be seen on the first slide. There is a primary concentration of tumors in the Free Hospital for Women ($N = 38$); Massachusetts General is next ($N = 21$); the Peter Bent Brigham is next ($N = 9$), and in the Children's Medical Center there were three tumors in the adolescent age range in those years. The only thing these data mean is that the patients were heavily concentrated in a specialty hospital for women which is what all of us would expect. Data on the admissions during that 10-year period for any of the four hospitals were not obtained; therefore the prevalence of these tumors in the general population, particularly in the two general hospitals, is not known, but presumably it is quite rare. The largest tumor in the series was a pseudomucinous cystadenoma which weighed about 7 kg. In this series of 72 tumors, there was one recorded death at the time the study was done. This occurred in a 19-year-old girl who had a malignant teratoma; she succumbed 1 year later. There were three kinds of information that one could gather from this study and we can discuss here today briefly. The first is the type and distribution of tumors that one encounters in this age group. Second are the clinical signs and symptoms in girls who had ovarian tumors in this study.

Third is whether the tumors found in adolescents differ in type from those found in children or from those in adults.

Let's address ourselves first to the type and distribution of tumors. The most common tumor in adolescence is the teratoma group. Actually, we classified them as teratoma-dermoids, and there were 23 cases in this classification which made up approximately 32 per cent of all the tumors found in the adolescent age group. Approximately a third of the tumors found in adolescent girls, at least in this study, fall in this classification. Of the 23 youngsters, one had a tumor that was malignant. One of the benign tumors had arrhenoblastoma elements in it, and a second one was a struma ovarii. For the benefit of the pediatricians in the group, a struma ovarii is a teratoma in which thyroid tissue is found. Actually, to qualify for the full meaning of this term, thyroid tissue should overgrow all the other elements of the tumor to become the predominant tissue. It is of some interest apparently that this tissue may be functionally active. Recently, in our adolescent inpatient unit, we had a girl with an ovarian tumor which was a teratoma-dermoid with thyroid tissue in it. Teratomas in general have been divided into teratomas and dermoid cysts. The histogenesis is identical, but some pathologists feel that there are points of difference. That is, the dermoid is a cystic tumor whereas the teratoma is a solid tumor. A dermoid cyst shows predominance of ectodermal elements, although occasionally endodermal or mesodermal elements are found. In the teratoma, all three of the cell types are found. The dermoid cyst is a benign tumor while the teratoma in general is a malignant tumor. About 25 per cent of the dermoids are considered to be bilateral. The teratomas are far less common than the dermoid and they are said to be proportionately more common in the young than is the dermoid. Our data did not particularly confirm this.

The second most frequent group of tumors in this series is cystadenoma (serous or pseudomucinous) of the ovaries. In this study, there were 14 cystadenomas, comprising approximately 20 per cent of the total number of cases. The pseudomucinous tumors of the ovaries are epithelial tumors which are filled with pseudomucinous-like material. They are large tumors, they are multilobulated, and they may undergo malignant degeneration.

Malignant degeneration is thought to occur in about 10 to 14 per cent. The serous cystadenoma, of which there were 5 in this particular series, is again an epithelial tumor of the ovary which is filled with cystic fluid which is rich in serum proteins. In general, they are not as large as a pseudomucinous tumor, are multiloculated, and are lobular. The serous cystadenofibroma, of which there were 8, is a serous cystadenoma in which there has been invagination of the epithelial lining of the tumor and the gland-like nature of this has become cystic.

There were 8 simple cysts and 5 corpus luteum cysts. Simple cysts are simply large simple cysts of the ovary, part of the normal physiological process, that for sometimes unclear reasons become large and tend to persist. There were 8 simple cysts and 5 examples of corpus luteum cysts which again are thought to be "a physiological" variation of the normal menstrual process. There were 4 parovarian cysts. Parovarian represents the sexual portion of the Wolffian body which is located between the tube and the hilum of the ovary. The vestigial tubes may become cystic; they rarely become large, and they are not malignant. There were 4 examples of this particular entity. They do produce symptoms on occasion by torsion. There were 3 examples of endometrioma. These tumors are essentially endometriosis of the ovaries. There was 1 fibroma. Fibromas are small; occasionally they may reach a large size; they are very dense and solid tumors. The fibroma, as I understand it, was the tumor found in the original description of Meigs' syndrome.

There was 1 thecal luteoma. The thecal luteomas fall in the granulosa cell, thecoma cell tumor group. These are tumors which have a common cell origin and a common hormonal effect. The hormonal effect is that of feminization or effects associated with the production of excessive estrogen. The granulosa cell tumor is derived from ovarian mesenchyme which has primary epithelial characteristics. It is endocrinely active, a feminizing estrogen producing tumor. The granulosa cell tumor rarely is found in pure cell type and may have small amounts of thecal cells as connective tissue cells in it. These tumors may be extremely small or they may be large. They are usually found during the reproductive period of life but they may be found in the prepuberty period where they cause precocious puberty. During the reproductive period, either in adolescence or in adult life, they may produce hypermenorrhagia; there may be normal menses associated with them, or there may be amenorrhea. In contrast, there is a thecoma which is a solid tumor of the ovary It is possibly derived from production by the ovarian mesenchyme of a connective tissue tumor which is endocrinely active in producing increased amounts of estrogen. The thecoma is rarely found in pure form, similar to the granulosa cell tumor, and it is common to have small numbers of granulosa cells in a thecoma.

With this as a background, there was in this series one thecal luteoma which is an endocrinely active tumor in which luteinization appears to have occurred. There is some evidence that luteinization is associated with the production of progesterone in these tumors, but it is the opinion of Novak that functionally such a term should not specifically imply progestational effect from this tumor and that the histological appearance in this instance does not automatically mean endocrine function usually associated with this cell type.

There was one dysgerminoma in the adolescent series. The dysgerminoma may be a small or large tumor of the ovary. It is one-third as frequent as the thecoma or the thecal cell tumors which makes it rather rare. It is a solid smooth tumor and tends to occur early in the life of a woman, that is, either before puberty, during adolescence or, in early reproductive life. For this reason those of us in adolescent medicine may have occasion to see a dysgerminoma. In general, it is biologically inert and its cell type resembles that of the testicles. Another name that has been used for dysgerminoma is seminoma. Approximately a third of them are said to be malignant.

There was 1 instance of a perineal inclusion cyst, 1 instance of a serous cystadenocarcinoma, and 1 embryonal cell carcinoma.

It might be worthwhile to discuss briefly for the sake of completeness, though we did not have an example in this series, an example of a masculinizing tumor of the ovary. The arrhenoblastoma is usually a small to modest size tumor and only on occasion does it become large. The clinical picture is that of amenorrhea and hirsutism, the latter developing over a period of time. The hirsutism involves the trunk as well as the face. I'm sure we'll hear a good deal more about that this afternoon from Dr. Greenblatt. Atrophy of the breasts, and roughening of the voice occurs; hypertrophy of the clitoris is noted, and on physical examination a tumor of the ovary may be palpated. This is a tumor of young women in their 20's and 20's; however, it has been reported during adolescence. It has a malignancy rate of approximately 25 per cent. This gets us through the rather boring recital of statistics. It does give us some idea of the probabilities that we might consider when a mass which is thought to be ovarian is present.

Are there any clinical findings which will indicate whether an ovarian tumor might be present, and, secondly, what kind of ovarian tumor is most likely? Clinical manifestations were correlated with the tumors under study. Rather than subgrouping, the tumors were considered as a group on their correlation with various clinical manifestations.

The most common symptom was abdominal pain (53.4 per cent) followed by menstrual disturbances (39 per cent) such as menorrhagia and dysmenorrhea. Nausea and vomiting were encountered in 27 per cent of the subjects. Vaginal mass or tenderness was present in 76 per cent of girls with rectal mass or tenderness noted in 63 per cent. Either a vaginal or a rectal examination will have a high probability of detecting an ovarian tumor in adolescent girls. An abdominal mass was palpable in 49 per cent and abdominal tenderness was elicited in 25 per cent of the girls. It is clear from these data that a thorough history and particularly the physical examination will be effective in detecting ovarian tumors in adolescent girls.

Is there any difference between the tumors found in adolescents and those found in adult women or children? For comparison with children's tumors, we took a report by Reiss and Koop[3] from Children's Hospital in Philadelphia who reported some 26 tumors seen in children under the age of 12 between the years of 1947 and 1961. For the adult group, we took a series of tumors reported by Galt and associates in which there were 317 consecutive ovarian tumors in adult women.[1] I took the liberty of shuffling the reported cases a little so that comparisons could be made. During adolescence the most common tumors were of the teratoma-dermoid cyst group which comprised about one-third of the tumors. In children, the teratoma-dermoid was the highest group of tumors which comprised about 45 per cent of their reported cases. In adult women, the teratomas comprised approximately 10 per cent. It would appear then that the teratoma-dermoid group is most apt to be found in younger children, with decreased frequency in adolescents, and least frequency in the adult women. Thus adolescents appear to be in a transitional period in regard to teratoma-dermoid tumors.

The next most common group of tumor in the adolescent was the cystadenoma which comprised some 30 per cent of tumors. In the children's series, there was only one cystadenoma out of 26. In the adult series the number of cystadenomas comprised almost 50 per cent of all the tumors. It would appear then that the cystadenomas are relatively infrequent in childhood, become more frequent during adolescence, and appear to make up the bulk of the adult tumor group.

In regard to carcinoma of the ovary, in the children's group there was only one that could be classified as carcinoma; in the adolescent tumors possibly 3 per cent could be classified as carcinomas, whereas in the adult group approximately 30 per cent of the tumors were carcinomatous. In children and in adolescents, carcinoma of the ovary is relatively rare; it begins to appear in adolescence, while during adult life it comprises a significant portion of ovarian tumors.

In regard to feminizing tumors of the ovaries, such as granulosa or theca-cell tumors, there were 3 out of 26, or approximately 10 per cent, in children. In adolescents there was one granulosa cell thecoma tumor, while in the adult series there were 13 out of 317 tumors. There were no arrhenoblastomas in either the children's or adolescents' series and one out of 317 in Galt's series.

These data would indicate that there are some differences between the frequency of certain kinds of tumors in adolescents as compared to children and adults, and there are some similarities. It would appear that these data taken in their entirety could be helpful in determining whether an ovarian tumor is present in an adolescent girl and what kind of tumor might be expected.

REFERENCES

1. Gault, E. W., Balafubrahmanyan, M., Thomas, E., Isaiah, P., Aleyamma, M. T., and Susheela, K. K.: Ovarian tumors; analysis of 317 consecutive ovarian tumors examined in pathology department of Christian Medical College, Vellore, 1943–1953. Indian J. M. Sc., 8: 522, 1954.
2. Heald, F., Craig, J., and Ming, P.: *Ovarian Tumors in Adolescent Girls,* in press.
3. Reiss, R., and Koop, C.: Ovarian tumors in infants and children. J. Pediat., 60: 96, 1962.

7

Hirsutism*

*Virendra B. Mahesh, Ph.D., D.Phil. and
Robert B. Greenblatt, M.D.*

The problem of hirsutism has attracted considerable attention in the past and still continues to offer a challenge because of the lack of suitable methods for its cure. Although marked hirsutism is comparatively easy to observe, it is often difficult to distinguish a mildly hirsute patient from a normal woman because of the wide spectrum of individual variation in the amount and distribution of facial and body hair in normal women. The cause of hirsutism may be genetic or endocrine.

GENETIC FACTORS

In evaluating genetic factors, due consideration should be given to racial factors. Caucasian populations, both male and female, have a larger surface area of sexual hair distribution than do Mongolians. Within the same race, there appears in many cases a familial tendency towards hirsutism. This may be due to increased end organ sensitivity or individual predisposition to hair growth. It may be of interest to consider the hair distribution on the extremities and dorsum of a girl aged 5 shown in Figure 7.1A and B. Such hairiness is probably an atavistic manifestation rather than a problem of endocrine origin and may persist into adulthood in some and disappear in others. In rare instances, a

* From the Department of Endocrinology, Medical College of Georgia, Augusta, Georgia.

78   ADOLESCENT GYNECOLOGY

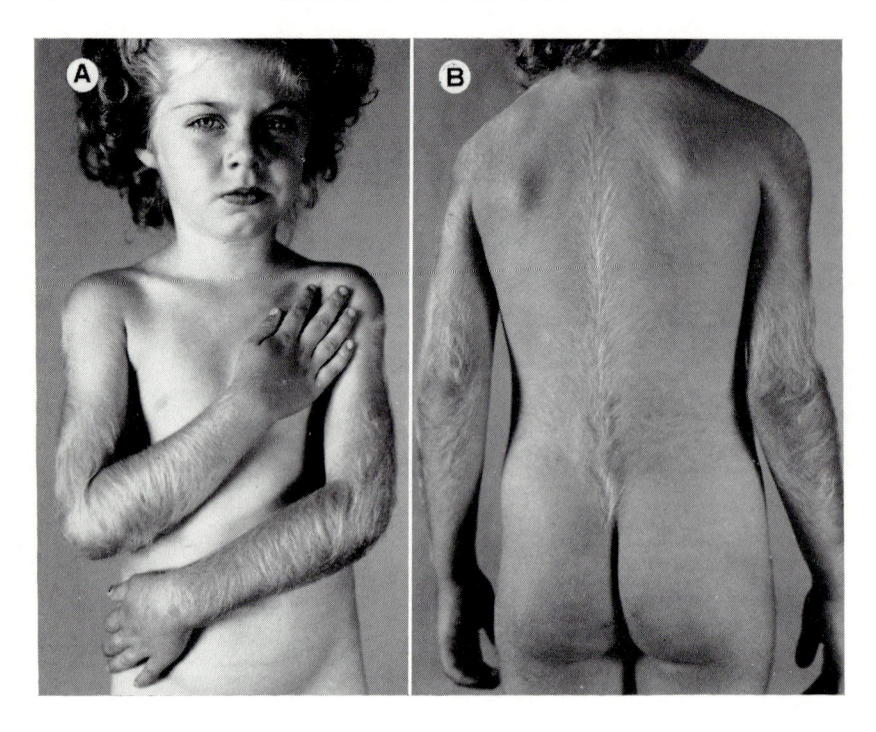

Fig. 7.1, *A* and *B*. Atavistic hypertrichosis in a child aged 5. (From Greenblatt, *The Hirsute Female*. Charles C Thomas, Springfield, Illinois.)

child with hypothyroidism has a similar degree of hairiness responsive to thyroid medication.[44]

ENDOCRINE FACTORS

General Considerations

Clinical experience with patients having pituitary, adrenal, or gonadal failure as well as those with adrenal and/or gonadal hyperfunction or tumors has demonstrated conclusively that the growth of sexual hair is regulated by androgen secretion. This impression has been borne out amply by the growth of sexual hair in patients given androgens for replacement therapy and by the development of iatrogenic hirsutism by excessive androgen administration. Due to the close relationship between androgens and hirsutism, considerable emphasis has been laid on the androgen secretion of a patient in the evaluation of hirsutism.

STUDY OF URINARY STEROID EXCRETION PATTERNS FOR EVALUATING ADRENAL AND OVARIAN ANDROGENS

For quite some time the myth has existed that 17-ketosteroid determinations on relatively crude urinary extracts are a measure of circulating androgens of the body. The magnitude of interfering material in such extracts is so great that the determinations are only of value in ascertaining gross changes in the secretion of steroids as observed in adrenal failure or in the presence of adrenal and gonadal tumors. Chromatographic separation and purification followed by individual estimation of various urinary steroids has offered a much more reliable procedure for the evaluation of androgen secretion. In spite of this, the origin of excessive androgens is still difficult to evaluate because the androgens secreted by the adrenals and the ovaries are identical or closely related structurally and they give rise to the same urinary metabolites. The estimation of various urinary steroids before and after adrenal suppression with dexamethasone yields a rough measure of adrenal and ovarian androgen secretion.[41] In our laboratory 45 hirsute patients were studied. They could be divided into 4 groups on the basis of their urinary steroid excretion pattern (Fig. 7.2). Group 1 consisted of 6 patients with elevations both in the 11-oxygenated and 11-deoxy-17-ketosteroids. The 7 patients in Group 2 had elevation only in the 11-oxygenated 17-ketosteroids, particularly 11-hydroxy-androsterone. Group 3 consisted of 18 patients with elevated 11-deoxy-17-ketosteroids, and Group 4 consisted of 14 patients with normal values in all the steroid fractions examined.

Urinary 11-oxygenated-17-ketosteroids, with very rare exceptions, are metabolites of compounds of adrenal origin, such as cortisol and 11β-hydroxy-Δ^4-androstenedione. This steroid fraction was elevated in both Group 1 and Group 2. Statistical analysis by Duncan's multiple range analysis showed that this elevation was highly significant (P = 0.01). These observations indicate that the excessive secretion of androgens in patients in Group 1 and Group 2 is principally of adrenal origin. Further support of this hypothesis is obtained by a satisfactory suppression of these elevated levels of steroids as compared with the normal on dexamethasone administration (Fig. 7.3).

Patients in Group 3 had significant elevation in only the 11-

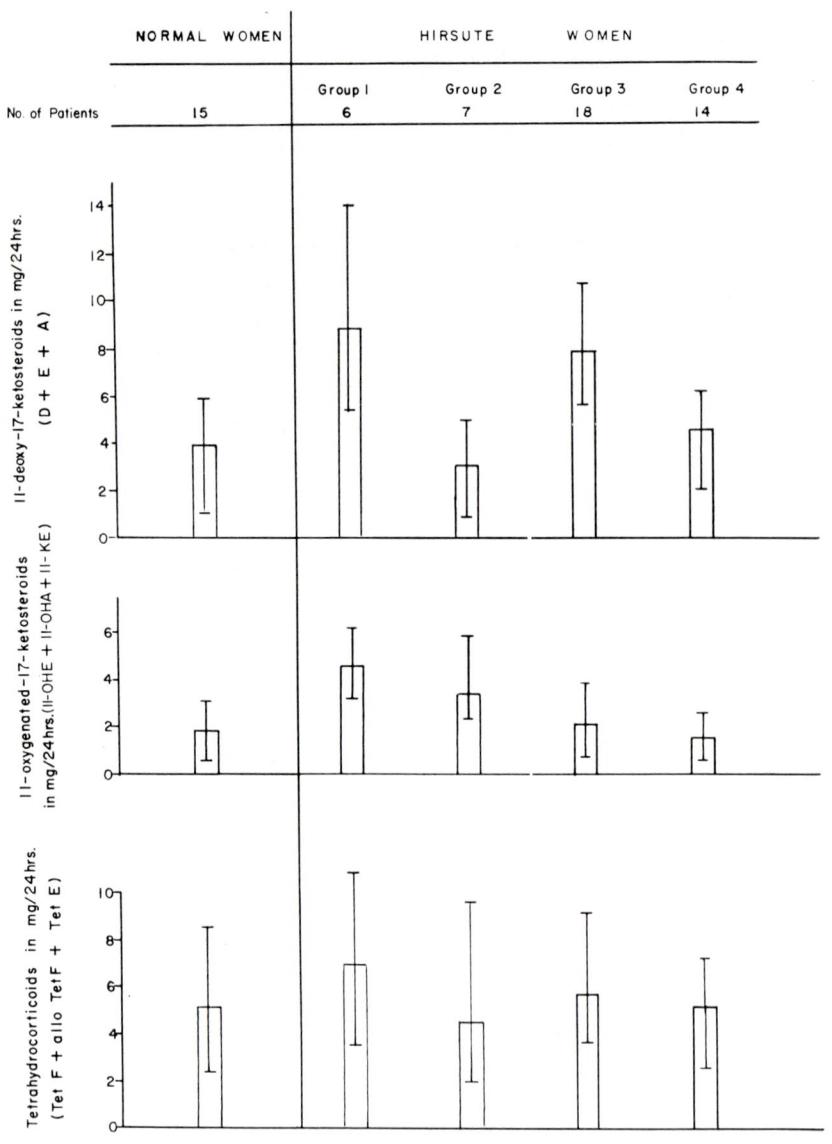

FIG. 7.2. Urinary steroid excretion patterns in normal and hirsute women. The hirsute women are divided in 4 groups based on urinary steroid excretion. Group 1 had elevations in both 11-deoxy and 11-oxygenated-17-ketosteroids; Group 2 had elevation only in the 11-oxygenated-17-ketosteroids, whereas, Group 3 had elevated 11-deoxy-17-ketosteroids. In Group 4 all values were within normal limits.

deoxy-17-ketosteroid fraction (P = 0.01). These steroids could arise either from the adrenal or from the ovary. This group was divided in three subgroups (Group 3a, 3b, and 3c) based on the patients' response to dexamethasone.

When adrenal suppression was attempted by dexamethasone administration, the mean value for the residual 11-deoxy-17-ketosteroids in milligrams per 24 hr. was found to be 1.2 in Group 3a (5 patients) and 3.9 in Group 3b (10 patients) as compared to 1.0 in normal women (Fig. 7.4). The difference in Group 3b as compared to normal and hirsute women in Group 3a is highly significant (P values in Students' T test and Duncan's multi range analysis, 0.01). These findings suggest that in Group 3a the elevation of 11-deoxy-17-ketosteroids is of adrenal origin, whereas in Group 3b they may be of ovarian origin. That the excessive ketosteroid production in Group 3b is ovarian in origin is supported by an almost complete reduction of these values when ovarian function is suppressed by the administration of stilbestrol. It may be argued that this fall is not due to ovarian suppression but further suppression of adrenals with dexamethasone. Although this possibility cannot be completely ruled out, it is somewhat unlikely, as adrenal suppression appeared to be adequate as judged from the suppression of 11-oxygenated-17-ketosteroids and tetrahydrocorticoids before the administration of stilbestrol. Confirmation of the ovarian origin of excessive androgen in Group 3b is obtained by a significant fall of these steroids after wedge-resection of the ovary (P = 0.01). Furthermore, when the ovaries of patients of Group 3b were stimulated with human pituitary follicle stimulating hormone (FSH) while the adrenals were suppressed, there was a marked rise in urinary 11-deoxy-17-ketosteroids as compared to only small increases in the other groups studied (Fig. 7.5).[35, 37, 39, 40] Further confirmation of excessive secretion of androgens by the polycystic ovaries was obtained by the isolation of large quantities of dehydroepiandrosterone and/or Δ^4-androstenedione from ovarian tissue as well as ovarian venous blood.[36, 39, 40]

Increased secretion of urinary 17-ketosteroids in hirsutism has been reported by several investigators and the adrenals were implicated in almost all the cases.[6, 8, 18, 20, 22, 23, 26, 32, 45] Although ovarian extracts were shown to have androgen activity in 1925[9] and a decrease in urinary androsterone was demonstrated after

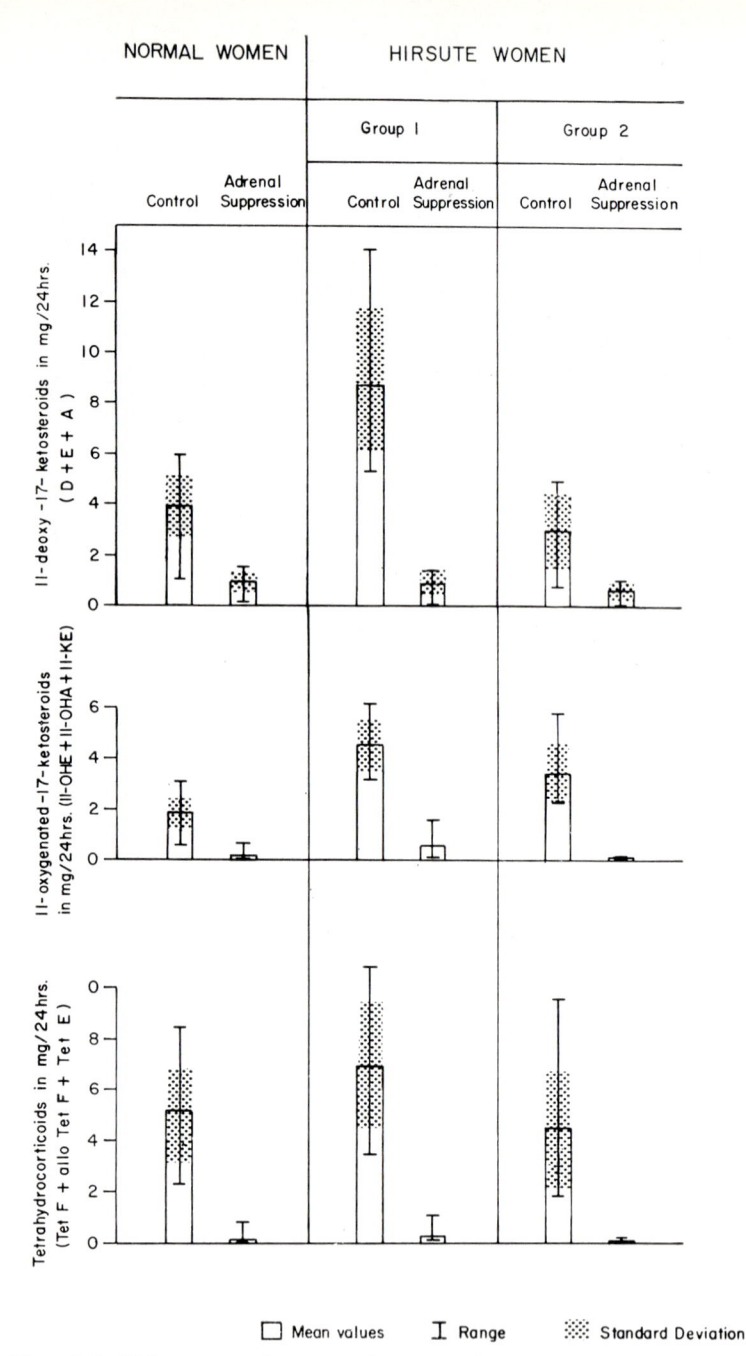

FIG. 7.3. Urinary 11-deoxy-17-ketosteroids, 11-oxygenated-17-ketosteroids and tetrahydrocorticoids in normal women and 2 groups of hirsute women. Group 1 (6 patients) had elevations in both 11-deoxy-17-ketosteroids and 11-oxygenated-17-ketosteroids (P = 0.01). Group 2 (7 patients) had elevated levels of only 11-oxygenated-17-ketosteroids (P = 0.05), particularly 11-hydroxyandrosterone (P = 0.01).

bilateral ovariectomy in 1940,[13] the contribution to significant androgen production by the ovaries in hirsutism was demonstrated by one of us for the first time in 1953.[23] A hirsute woman with functional uterine bleeding, polycystic ovaries, and adenocanthoma of the endometrium was found to have elevated 17-ketosteroids that showed only moderate lowering on cortisone but a marked reduction after bilateral oophorectomy (Fig. 7.6). The adrenal suppression test as shown by the above mentioned studies (Figs. 7.3 to 7.6) appears to be of considerable value in differentiating between androgen of adrenal and ovarian origin. Poor depression of 17-ketosteroids after adrenal suppression in patients with the Stein-Leventhal syndrome has been reported earlier by our group as well as by other investigators.[2, 21, 26, 29, 37, 39, 40, 41, 43, 46] An elevation in secretion rates of dehydroepiandrosterone and/or Δ^4-androstenedione and poor depression of urinary 17-ketosteroids after adrenal suppression in patients with Stein-Leventhal syndrome has also been reported.[33] An increase in urinary 17-ketosteroids and ketogenic steroids after sheep and human pituitary FSH administration was observed by Keetall and associates[30] and Gemzell and associates;[19] however, the source of the 17-ketosteroid precursors was not well established. The stimulation of ovarian androgen secretion after the administration of human chorionic gonadotropins has also been reported.

Considerable difficulty was experienced in trying to classify 3 hirsute patients in Group 3c (Fig. 7.7). An average fall of 5.7 mg. per 24 hr. was observed in the 11-deoxy-17-ketosteroid fraction after dexamethasone was administered. An average fall of 7.0 mg. per 24 hr. was observed in Group 1 and 5.7 in Group 3a under similar conditions. Both these groups appeared to have an adrenal hyperfunction. The fall in 11-deoxy-17-ketosteroids in normal women and those thought to have an ovarian disorder was considerably smaller. An adrenocorticotropic hormone (ACTH) stimulation test was performed on 2 of the 3 patients of Group 3c and an abnormal response was observed. After dexamethasone administration, the 11-deoxy-17-ketosteroids remained elevated as compared to the normal, whereas 11-oxy-

---

All patients showed good suppression after dexamethasone administration as compared to the normal. (From Mahesh, et al.: J. Clin. Endocrinol., *24:* 1283, 1964.)

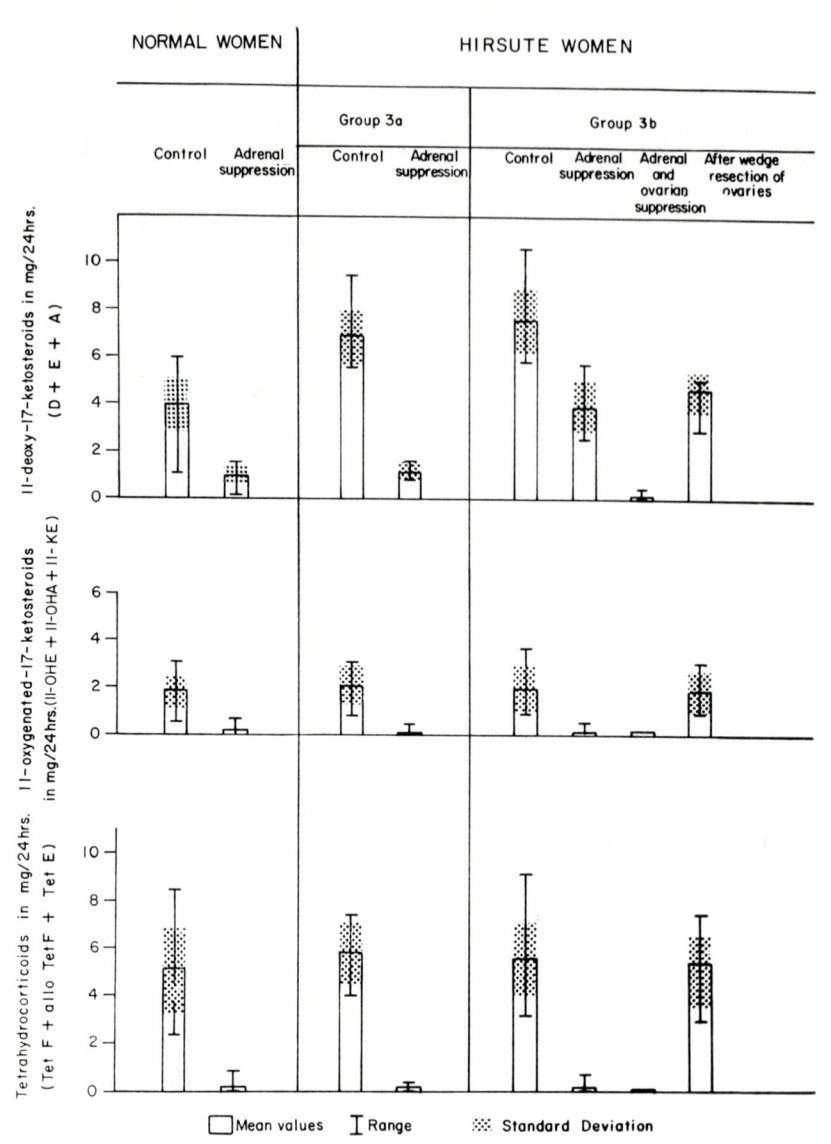

FIG. 7.4. Urinary steroid excretion pattern in hirsute patients in Group 3 shows elevation in the 11-deoxy-17-ketosteroid fraction (P = 0.01). On dexamethasone administration, the depression of 11-deoxy-17-ketosteroids was poor in Group 3b as compared to normal women and hirsute women in Group 3a (P = 0.01). Administration of stilbestrol brought about a further decrease in this fraction in Group 3b. Wedge-resection of the ovaries was carried out on 5 patients in Group 3b and a significant fall in 11-deoxy-17-ketosteroids was noted 3 months after the operation. (From Mahesh, et al.: J. Clin. Endocrinol., 24: 1283, 1964.)

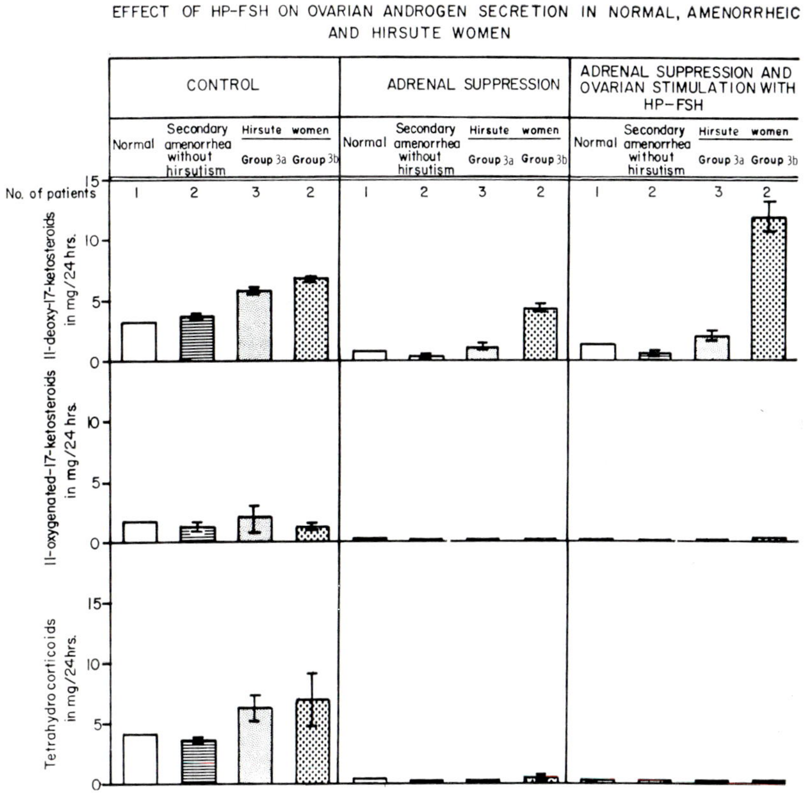

FIG. 7.5. Note poor depression of 11-deoxy-17-ketosteroids on adrenal suppression and a marked increase in these steroids after ovarian stimulation with human pituitary follicle stimulating hormone in Group 3b as compared to a normal subject, patients with secondary amenorrhea without hirsutism, and patients in Group 3a. (From Mahesh, et al.: J. Clin. Endocrinol., *24:* 1293, 1964.)

genated-17-ketosteroids and tetrahydrocorticoids were well suppressed. In 2 patients, these 11-deoxy-17-ketosteroid levels were suppressed with estrogens. These observations suggest both adrenal and ovarian involvement. This finding appears to be in agreement with the clinical observation that some patients require both adrenal suppression and wedge-resection for restoration of cyclical ovulatory menses.

In Group 4, 11 hirsute patients showed a normal steroid excretion pattern (Fig. 7.8). The response to adrenal suppression with dexamethasone was also within the normal range. The cause of

MARKEDLY HIRSUTE FEMALE WITH AMENORRHEA - MENORRHAGIA SYNDROME
w. f. 28, (N.H.)

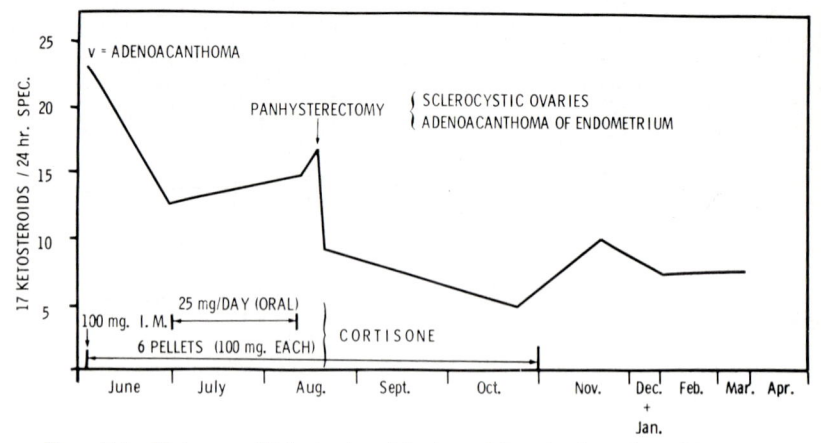

Fig. 7.6. Urinary 17-ketosteroids in a hirsute female with amenorrhea and menorrhagia before and after cortisone treatment and bilateral oophorectamy. Although there was a depression of 17-ketosteroids on cortisone treatment, further depression was observed after the removal of the ovaries. (From Greenblatt, Am. J. Obst. & Gynec., 66: 700, 1953.)

hirsutism or the etiology whether adrenal or ovarian in these patients is undetermined. In Group 4, 3 patients presented a problem. The 11-deoxy-17-ketosteroid levels were very slightly elevated, whereas the other steroids were within the normal range. The levels of the residual 11-deoxy-17-ketosteroids after adrenal suppression were found to be slightly above normal levels and between those found in Group 3a and Group 3b. It is, therefore, difficult to decide whether they belong to Group 3a or 3b or 4.

END-ORGAN SENSITIVITY TO ANDROGENS

The cause of hirsutism in Group 4 remains obscure. The development of methods for the determination of plasma testosterone levels and the reports of elevated plasma testosterone in virilism offered a shortlived hope that plasma testosterone levels would be the ultimate method for diagnosis in hirsutism.[7, 12, 15, 16, 27, 47] In a large number of cases of hirsutism, the plasma testosterone levels are found within normal limits, and no rational explanation for the hirsuties based on our present state of knowledge is available. Testosterone production rate has been also em-

URINARY STEROID EXCRETION PATTERN IN HIRSUTE WOMEN WITH PROBABLE MIXED ADRENAL AND OVARIAN HYPERFUNCTION

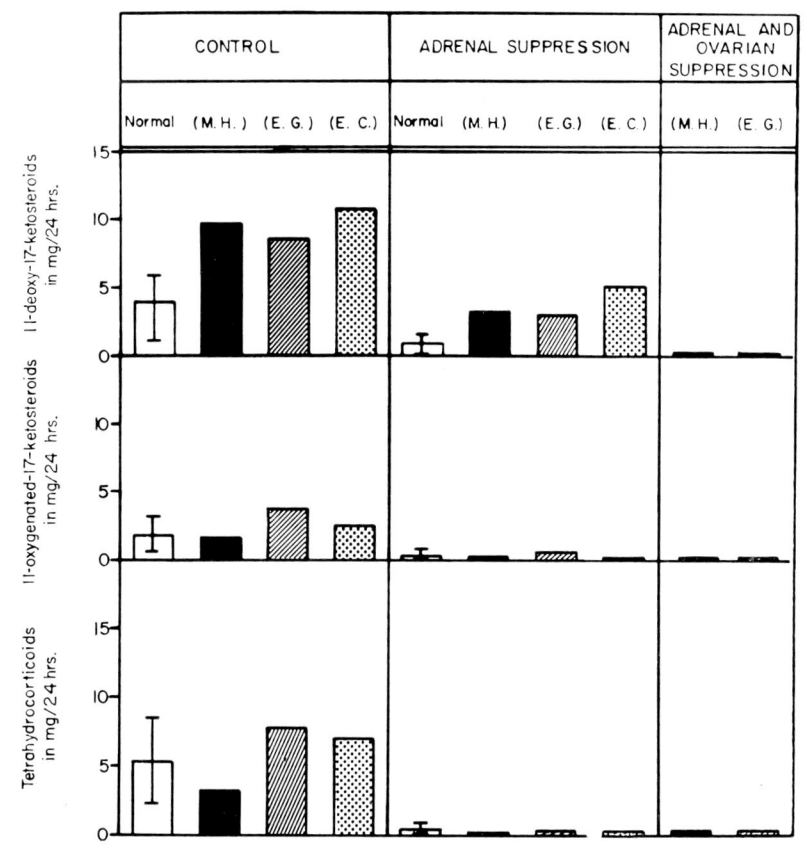

FIG. 7.7. Urinary steroid excretion pattern in 3 patients in Group 3c. Although there was a significant reduction in the elevated levels of 11-deoxy-17-ketosteroids after adrenal suppression, the levels remained high in comparison to the normal. They were reduced by ovarian suppression.

ployed by several investigators. It should, however, be borne in mind that testerone may be synthesised in the body by the peripheral conversion of precursors like dehydroepiandrosterone and Δ^4-androstenedione as shown by Mahesh and Greenblatt[34] in 1962. This observation has been confirmed by several investigators.[3, 51, 53] Furthermore, precursors like dehydroepiandrosterone may be converted directly to testosterone glucuronoside without circulating as free testosterone.[31] Therefore, testosterone produc-

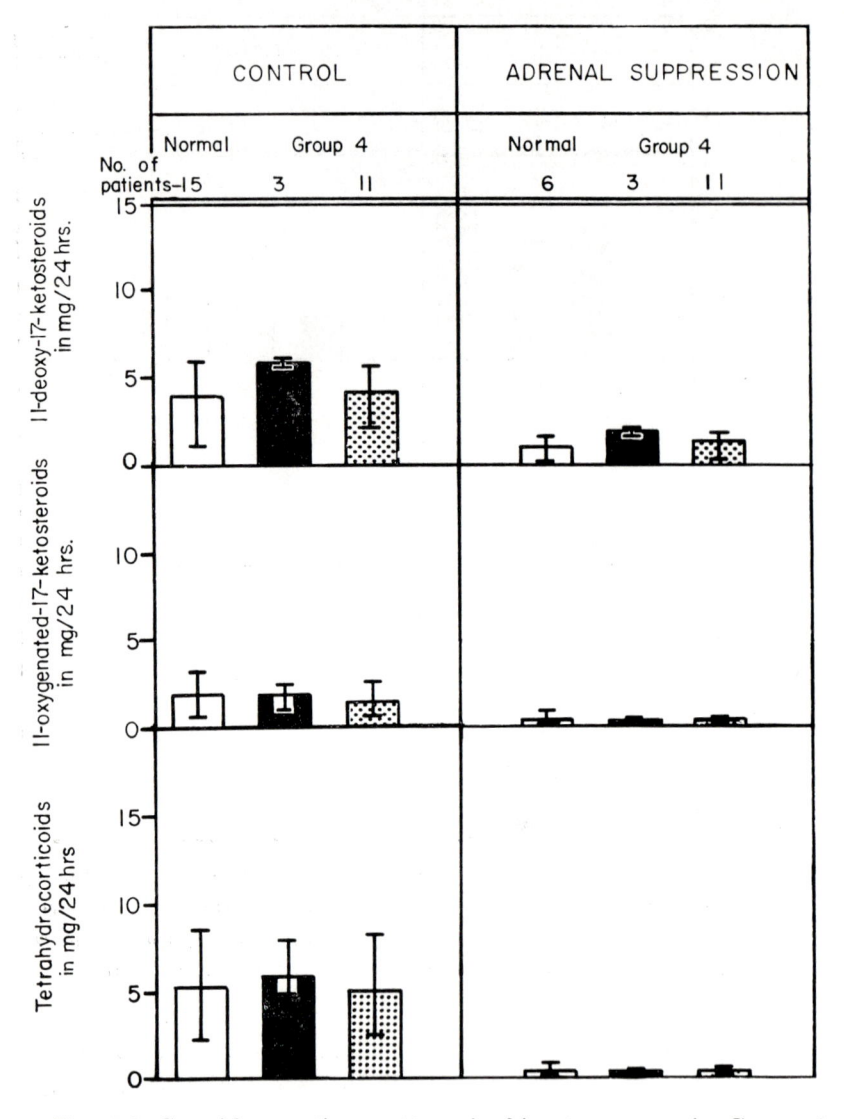

FIG. 7.8. Steroid excretion pattern in hirsute women in Group 4. Three of the patients showed only slight increase in 11-deoxy-17-ketosteroids and were difficult to classify. The remaining 11 patients showed a normal steroid excretion pattern.

tion rates do not reflect either the secretion or level of physiologically active testosterone circulating in the plasma.

The failure to detect excessive androgen production in patients in Group 4 may well be due to the limitations of experimental techniques. Nevertheless due emphasis must be placed on differences in end-organ sensitivity. The relatively poor end-organ sensitivity to androgens in the growth of sexual hair in Mongolians as compared to Caucasians has already been mentioned. Patients with breast cancer who have been treated with massive doses of androgens show a wide variation in hair growth, and this appears to provide additional indirect evidence for differences in end-organ sensitivity to androgens. Renewed attention is drawn to the importance of end-organ sensitivity in the syndrome of testicular feminization by the recent demonstration that the gonads secrete physiologically significant levels of androgens, and that the lack of sexual hair growth is due to failure of end-organ response to androgens.[17, 38, 42, 49]

Endocrine Disorders Associated with Hirsutism

STEIN-LEVENTHAL SYNDROME

The Stein-Leventhal syndrome was described originally by Stein and Leventhal in 1935 and is characterized by the association of hirsutism, obesity, secondary amenorrhea, and bilaterally enlarged polycystic ovaries.[50] All patients with the Stein-Leventhal syndrome may not be hirsute or obese. Furthermore, polycystic ovaries are found in many other conditions not associated with the Stein-Leventhal syndrome. Therefore, it becomes apparent that the clinical symptomotalgy of the Stein-Leventhal syndrome may arise from several different etiologies. The evaluation of the androgen secretion by the adrenals and ovaries, using methods of adrenal suppression and ovarian stimulation with human pituitary FSH, has already been mentioned in this article. These studies show that, although in the majority of cases the Stein-Leventhal syndrome is an ovarian defect, an identical clinical picture can also be obtained in adrenal disorders.[35, 39, 41] If the etiology is ovarian, wedge-resection of the ovaries is generally found to be most fruitful. In adrenal disorders, adrenal suppression is beneficial. Occasionally adrenal and ovarian suppression followed by electrolysis has yielded excellent results for the treatment of hirsutism in these cases. It should, however, be emphasized that the dangers of long term glucocorticoid treatment are many, and this type of treatment should only be administered by physicians oriented in endocrinology along with careful and rigorous periodical followup studies.

MALE PSEUDOHERMAPHRODITISM

Many patients with abdominal testes fall into the syndrome of "testicular feminization." In this syndrome, although the gonads are capable of secreting physiological levels of androgens and estrogens, there appears to be an end-organ insensitivity to androgens and thereby an absence of sexual hair growth.[17, 38, 42, 49] Occasionally there is an absence of the end-organ unresponsiveness in patients with abdominal testes and the patients are more or less virilized. During the last decade several cases of male pseudohermaphroditism have been described with one dysgenetic gonad (rudimentary gonadal streak) and a contralateral testis.[24, 25, 52, 56] A typical case history follows:

A 14-year-old individual, raised as a girl, was referred to us because of clitoral enlargement, amenorrhea, and absence of secondary sex characteristics. Her appearance suggested a diagnosis of male pseudohermaphroditism. From the history it was learned that the clitoris had been enlarging rapidly for the previous 2 years. Examination revealed a clitoris 4 cm. in length and about 2 cm. in diameter, which during tumescence measured about 6 cm. in length (Fig. 7.9). The urethral opening was in the position normal for a female and the vaginal introitus was small, barely admitting a finger. Urinary 17-ketosteroids were 3 mg., and urinary gonadotropins assayed more than 50 but less than 100 mouse units per 24 hr.

Laparotomy was performed. A uterus with bilateral fallopian tubes was found, but occupying the right adnexum was a testicle and the left, a rudimentary gonadal streak. Histological study of the excised testicle revealed fairly well developed tubular structures and interstitial Leydig cells (Fig. 7.10A). Biopsy of the rudimentary gonadal streak showed fibrous connective tissue stroma and some mesonephric rests lined by a low cuboidal epithelium (Fig. 7.10B). The penislike structure was removed. Histologically this was composed of the glans and corpora cavernosa.

Nuclear sex chromatin and chromosomal studies were carried

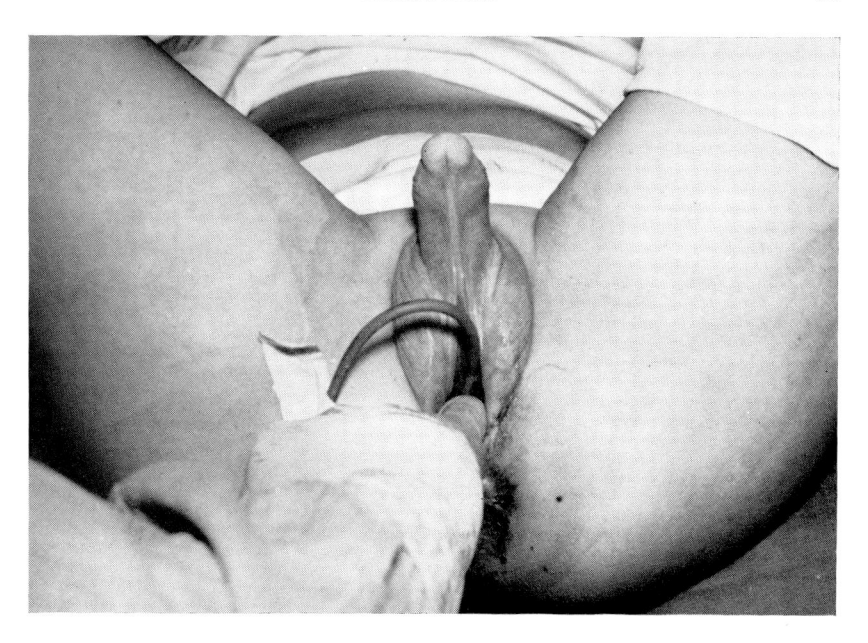

Fig. 7.9. Phallus-like organ and vaginal orifice below catheter inserted into urethra in 14-year-old female with a dysgenetic gonad and a contralateral testis. (From Greenblatt, et al.: J. A. M. A., *188:* 221, 1964.)

out. Negative oral and blood smears were found. Four samples of peripheral blood were cultured and a total of 65 cells in satisfactory metaphase were counted. Of these, 46 cells contained the normal 46 chromosomes and 15 cells had only 45 chromosomes. Three cells had 44 and one cell 47 chromosomes which were considered as probable technical artifacts. Karyotype analysis, according to the Denver classification, was performed on 11 cells containing 46 chromosomes and an XY chromosomal constitution was found. Four of the cells containing 45 chromosomes were karyotyped and an XO constitution was obtained. Therefore, the sex chromosome constitution in this patient was interpreted as a mosaic with an XO/XY pattern.

CONGENITAL ADRENAL HYPERPLASIA

The most frequent clinical manifestation of congenital adrenal hyperplasia in the female is virilization and pseudohermaphroditism. Marked clitoral enlargement with or without a urogenital sinus may be present. The urethral orifice may occupy a hy-

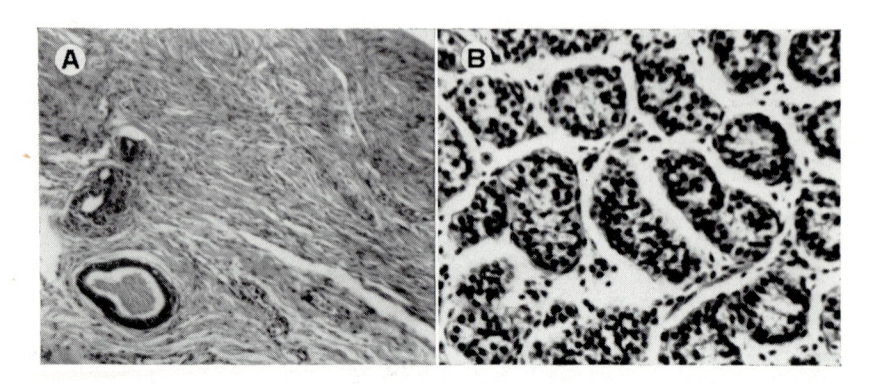

FIG. 7.10. *A*, histologic section of dysgenetic rudimentary gonadal streak. Note cortical tissue resembling ovarian stroma and remnants of mesonephros in hilus. *B*, histologic section of testis. Note immature seminiferous tubules. (From Greenblatt, et al.: J. A. M. A., *188:* 221, 1964.)

pospadiac position or open into the urogenital canal. The external os may serve as a cloaca for the urinary and genital passages. If the androgen excess from the adrenal occurs after a certain critical period of embryonic development the only abnormality at birth may be clitoral enlargement.

Clinically, at least three distinct types of congenital adrenal hyperplasia are known, and urinary pregnanetriol is elevated in all of these types. Congenital adrenal hyperplasia with virilization as the only clinical manifestation is called "uncomplicated" or "compensated" form. A case of this type was first reported in 1865 by de Crecchio.[10] Based on the presence of elevated levels of pregnanetriol and 17-ketosteroids in urine and their ready suppression with cortisone,[1, 5, 54] Jailer[28] postulated that the principal disorder in congenital adrenal hyperplasia was the failure of further hydroxylation of 17 α-hydroxyprogesterone to cortisol. This hypothesis was confirmed by Bongiovanni by demonstration of a 21-hydroxylase deficiency in the adrenals.[4] This enzymatic deficiency does not lead to a complete block in cortical synthesis. In an attempt to produce physiological levels of cortisol in the presence of a 21-hydroxylase deficiency, there is increased ACTH secretion by the pituitary with the production of abnormally large quantities of cortisol precursors and androgens. These excessive androgens are responsible for virilism. In the salt losing form of congenital adrenal hyperplasia the virilization is accompanied by vomiting, dehydration, and circulatory collapse similar to an Addisonian crisis. Although several different pathogeneses have been suggested, the current view is that the 21-hydroxylase deficiency is more complete, blocking aldosterone production and thus giving rise to the salt loss.[11, 14]

The hypertensive form of congenital adrenal hyperplasia was first described by Wilkins and associates[55] and Shepard and Clausen[48] who demonstrated that the vascular hypertension could be controlled by cortisone administration. The principal abnormality in this form of the syndrome appears to be a failure of the adrenal 11β hydroxylase. A typical case history follows:

W.M.F., a 15-year-old pseudohermaphrodite, had a male bodily habitus (Fig. 7.11A), hypertension (164/98 mg. Hg), amenorrhea, markedly enlarged clitoris, and a urogenital sinus. She had a female sex chromatin pattern and a castrate smear. Urinary 17-ketosteroids (70 mg. per 24 hr.), Allen test for dehydroepiandrosterone (15 to 30 mg. per 24 hr.), and pregnanetriol (5.4 mg. per 24 hr.) were elevated. Serum potassium was decreased (3.3 and 3.0 meq per liter); serum chlorides were elevated (109 and 113 mEq per liter); serum sodium was normal (138 and 143 μg. per liter). Intravenous hydrocortisone (100 mg. b.i.d. for 2 days) followed by prednisone (10 mg. orally t.i.d. for 8 days) produced satisfactory suppression of urinary 17-ketosteroids, pregnanetriol, and dehydroepiandrosterone (Fig. 7.12). Exploratory laparotomy revealed large polycystic ovaries. The patient was placed on maintenance therapy with hydrocortisone and potassium chloride. She showed gratifying progress and experienced her first spontaneous menstrual period after 3 months (Fig. 7.11B).

ADRENAL VIRILIZATION

Adrenal hyperfunction resulting in excessive secretion of androgens may result in virilization and hirsutism. Mention of adrenal disorders has already been made in connection with congenital adrenal hyperplasia and the Stein-Leventhal syndrome. In Cushing's syndrome due to adrenal hyperplasia or tumor, the excessive corticoid production may be accompanied by excessive androgens giving rise to hirsutism. Virilizing adrenal tumors may also be encountered in adolescent girls giving rise to extensive hirsutism. In general, the sudden onset of symptomatology, pres-

94   ADOLESCENT GYNECOLOGY

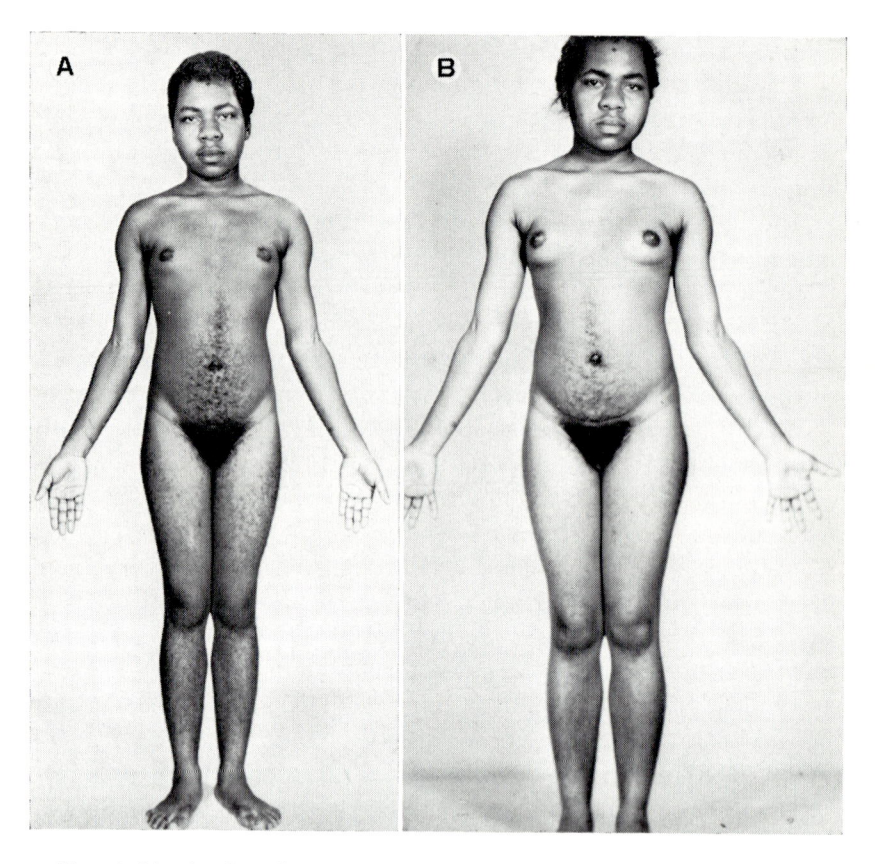

Fig. 7.11. *A*, female pseudohermaphrodite with hypertension. *B*, after cortisone therapy breast development and spontaneous menses occurred. (From Greenblatt, Recent Progr. in Hormone Res., *14:* 335, 1958.)

ence of moderate to highly elevated levels of urinary 17-ketosteroids that do not suppress adequately on dexamethasone administration, and absence of significant levels of urinary pregnanetriol are usually diagnostic. These criteria are not foolproof as in a small number of cases the adrenals may suppress well in the presence of a tumor. Presacral air insufflation studies are also useful in obtaining evidence for a tumor. A typical case history follows:

B.G.C., 17 years of age, complained of increasing hirsutism from age 13 onwards. She had experienced acne during the last 4 years and had had considerable voice change over a 2-year period. Menarche set in at 12 with painless menses occurring at 28 to 38

HIRSUTISM

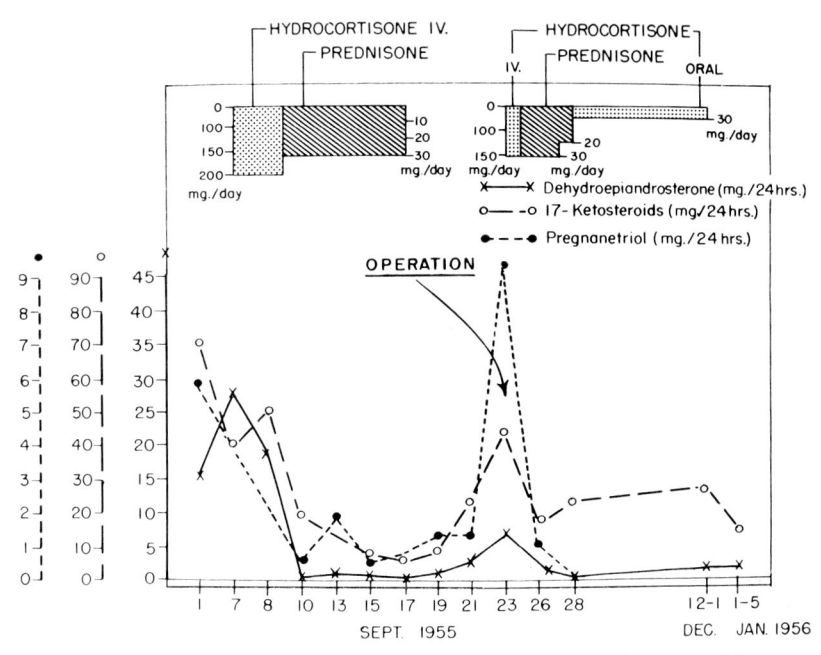

FIG. 7.12. Urinary dehydroepiandrosterone, 17-ketosteroids, and pregnanetriol in the female pseudohermaphrodite (Fig. 11A) before and after cortisone treatment. (From Greenblatt, Recent Progr. in Hormone Res., *14:* 335, 1958.)

day intervals. Physical examination revealed marked hairiness of face, chest, abdomen, and extremities (Fig. 7.13A and B). The breasts were well developed and the clitoris moderately enlarged. No abnormalities were found in the recto-pelvic examination. The sex chromatin and the chromosomal analysis were also of the normal female type. Presacral air insufflation suggested a tumor of the left adrenal.

Urinary 17-ketosteroids levels were found to be very high and could not be suppressed adequately by the administration of dexamethasone (2 mg. every 6 hr.) as judged by the 11-deoxy-17-ketosteroids (Table 7.1). It is of interest to note that interferring substances in urine prevented estimation of 17-ketogenic steroids and at the same time gave the mistaken impression of a remarkable fall in total 17-ketosteroids. This serves as an example of the limitations of the total 17-ketosteroid determinations on crude urinary extracts. Urinary pregnanetriol was within normal limits indicating the absence of congenital adrenal hyperplasia.

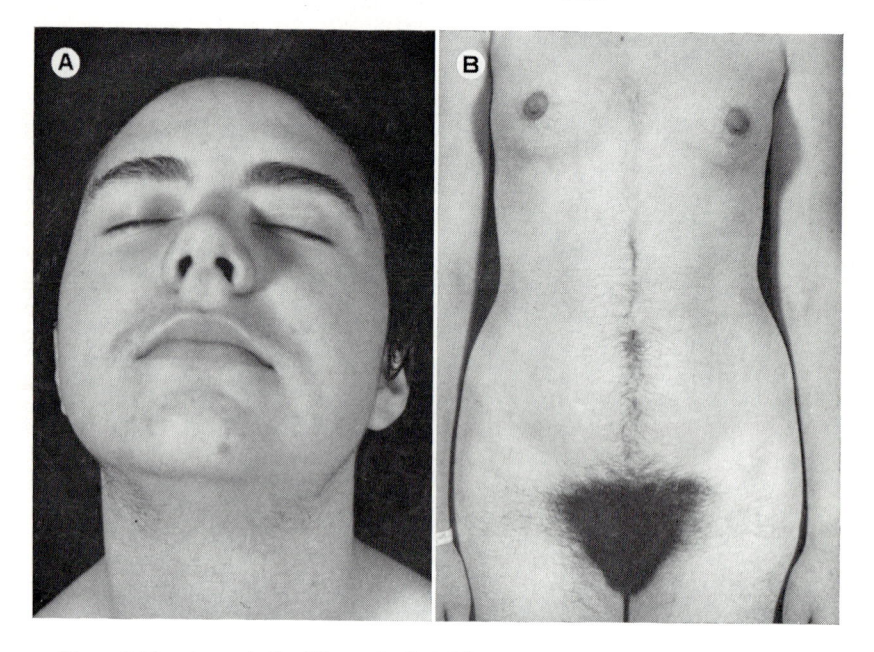

Fig. 7.13, *A* and *B*. Note facial hirsuties and distribution of hair on chest and abdomen in a 17-year-old patient with an adrenal tumor.

At laparotomy a tumor of the left adrenal was found and removed (Fig. 7.14), which histologically was diagnosed as an adenoma. The patient appears well a year after surgery. Urinary steroids are within the normal range. The hirsutism is somewhat lessened and the menstrual pattern remains the same except for pain associated with them.

OVARIAN TUMORS

The most common type of masculinizing ovarian tumor is the arrhenoblastoma and less common are Leydig or Hilar cell tumors and gynandroblastomas. Usually the patient presents with a history of recent onset of hirsutism, amenorrhea, voice changes, and enlargement of the clitoris. Generally a mass is palpable in the adnexal region. Urinary 17-ketosteroids in most instances are within normal limits because such tumors are known to produce significant amounts of testosterone. The level of testosterone produced, although quantitatively small as compared to other weaker androgens, nevertheless has enough physiological activity to account for the symptoms. A typical case history follows:

HIRSUTISM

TABLE 7.1
Urinary Steroid Excretion in an 18-Year-Old Girl with Adrenal Tumor Before and After Adrenal Suppression and After Removal of the Tumor

Medication	Routine 17-Ketosteroids	17-Ketogenic Steroids	11-Deoxy-17-Ketosteroids*	11-Oxy- + 17-Ketosteroids*	Tetrahydrocorticoids*	Pregnanetriol
	mg./24 hr.	mg./24 hr.	mg./24 hr.	mg./24 hr.	mg./24 hr.	mg./24 hr.
May 1964						
Control	136.8	†	22.4	2.7	6.8	1.4
Control	132.8	†	21.2	3.1	6.4	1.4
Dexamethasone, 2 mg. every 6 hr.						
3rd day	18.0	†	18.4	0.6	0.4	—
4th day	21.7	†	20.1	0.7	0.4	—
Tumor removed in June 1964						
April 1965						
Control	8.0	4.2				
July 1965						
Control	8.1	3.7				

* Normal values of 11-deoxy-17-ketosteroids 1.1 to 5.9 mg. per 24 hr., 11-oxy-17-ketosteroids 0.6 to 3.1 mg. per 24 hr., and tetrahydrocorticoids 2.3 to 8.5 mg. per 24 hr. From Mahesh and associates.[41]

† Interferring substances prevented estimation of 17-ketogenic steroids.

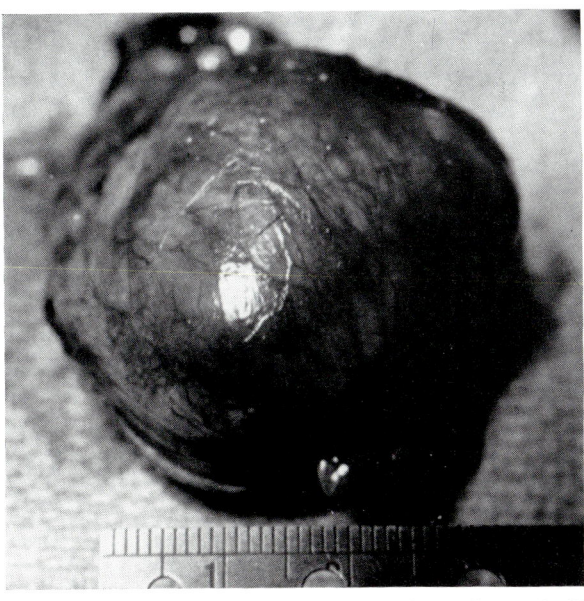

FIG. 7.14. Tumor of the left adrenal of patient shown in Figure 7.13. It was diagnosed histologically as an adenoma.

98   ADOLESCENT GYNECOLOGY

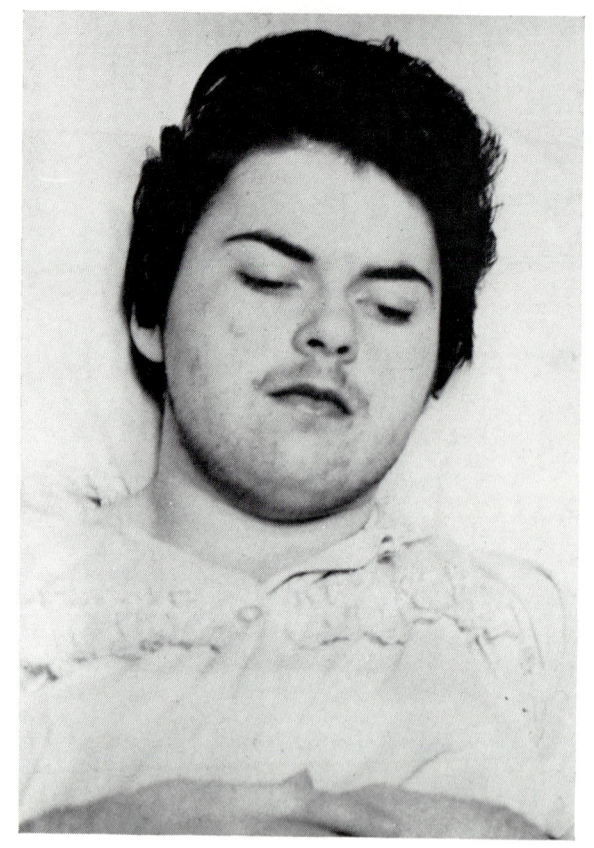

Fig. 7.15. Marked hypertrichosis in an 18-year-old harboring a virilizing ovarian tumor.

A.P., 18 years of age, was referred to us because of increasing hirsutism, enlargement of clitoris, and voice changes over a period of 1 year (Fig. 7.15). Menarche occurred at 12 with irregular menses for 2 years followed by amenorrhea. The breasts were rather small and vaginal cytology was of the castrate type. On rectal examination, a left adnexal mass was palpable, and a diagnosis of arrhenoblastoma was entertained. Urinary 17-ketosteroids were within normal limits (7.1 and 9.9 mg. per 24 hr.) as were the 17-ketogenic steroids, pregnanediol, and pregnanetriol. At laparotomy a cystic tumor, 11.5 cm. in diameter, was removed (Fig. 7.16). The histological diagnosis was arrhenoblastoma (Fig. 7.17). Spontaneous painful menses have recurred at regular in-

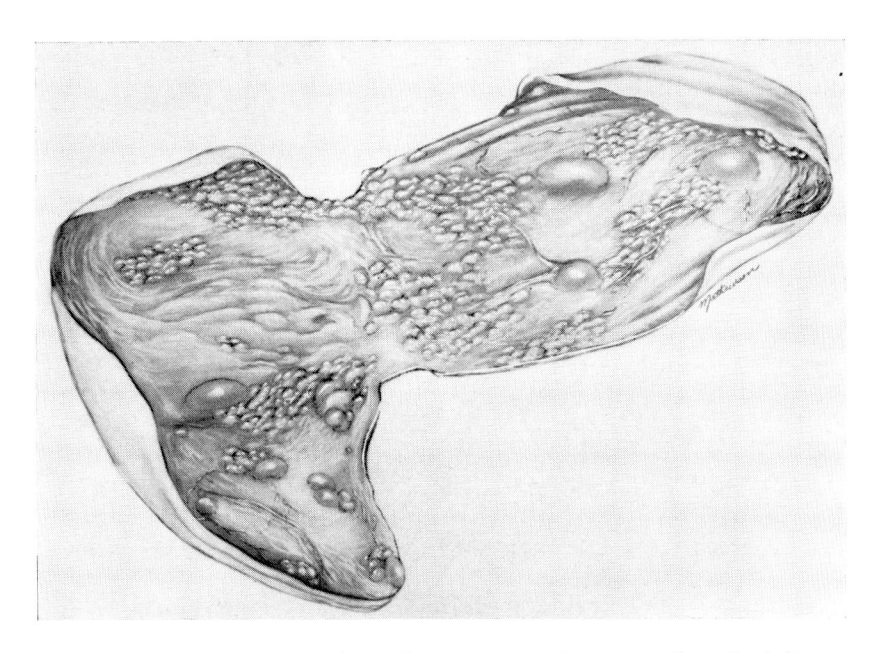

FIG. 7.16. Artist's drawing of opened cystic tumor found at laparotomy in patient (Fig. 7.15).

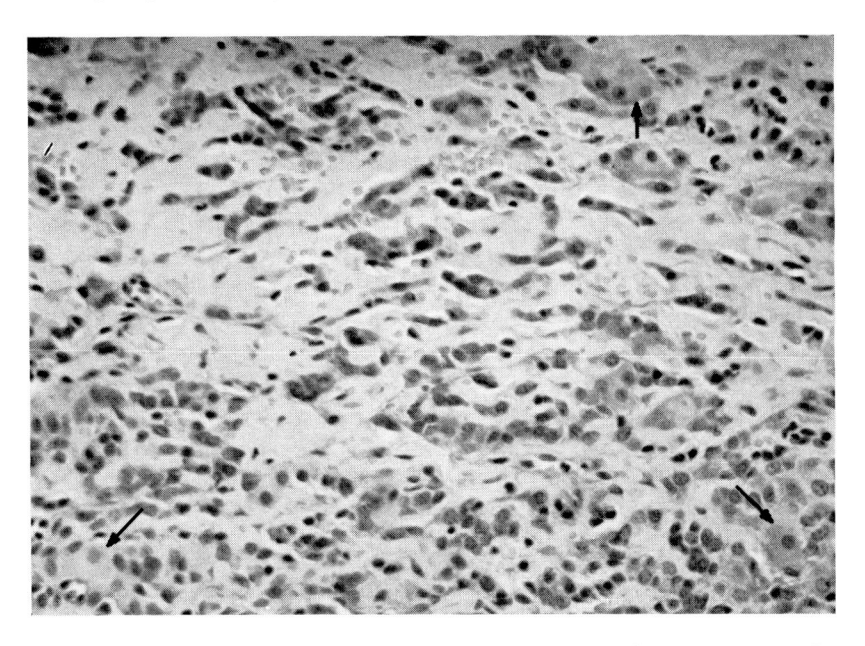

FIG. 7.17. Photomicrograph of histologic section through one of the nodules lining cystic tumor. Note fetal cord arrangement; *arrows* point to large pale Leydig-like cells.

tervals since surgery 4½ years ago. The breasts have enlarged and hirsutism has somewhat lessened.

REFERENCES

1. Bartter, F. C., Albright, F., Forbes, A. P., Leaf, A., Dempsey, E., and Carroll, E.: The effects of adrenocorticotropic hormone and cortisone in the adrenogenital syndrome associated with congenital adrenal hyperplasia. J. Clin. Invest., *30:* 237, 1951.
2. Baulieu, E. E., Mauvais-Jarvis, P., and Corpechot, C.: Steroid studies in a case of Stein-Leventhal syndrome with hirsutism. J. Clin. Endocrinol., *23:* 374, 1963.
3. Baulieu, E. E., and Robel, P.: ANDROST-5-ENE-3β, 17β-DIOL-17α-3H to testosterone-17α-3H and 5α and 5β-ANDROSTANE-3α, 17β-DIOL-17α-3H in vivo. Steroids, *2:* 111, 1963.
4. Bongiovanni, A. M.: In vitro hydroxylation of steroids by whole adrenal homogenates of beef, normal man, and patients with adrenogenital syndrome. J. Clin. Invest., *37:* 1342, 1958.
5. Bongiovanni, A. M., and Clayton, G. W., Jr.: Simplified method for the routine determination of pregnanediol and pregnanetriol in urine. Bull. Johns Hopkins Hosp., *94:* 180, 1954.
6. Brooks, R. V., and Prunty, F. T. G.: Patterns of steroid excretion in three types of post-pubertal hirsutism. J. Endocrinol., *21:* 263, 1960.
7. Burger, H. G., Kent, J. R., and Kellie, A. E.: Determination of testosterone in human peripheral and adrenal venous plasma. J. Clin. Endocrinol., *24:* 432, 1964.
8. Bush, I. E., and Mahesh, V. B.: Adrenocortical hyperfunction with sudden onset of hirsutism. J. Clin. Endocrinol., *18:* 1, 1959.
9. Champy, C., and Kritch, N.: Muco-elastic tissue of cock's comb a reagent for sexual hormone. Compt. Rend. Soc. Biol., *92:* 683, 1925.
10. de Crecchio, L.: Sopra un caso di apparenze virili in una donna. Morgagni, *7:* 151, 1865.
11. Degenhart, H. J., Visser, H. K. A., Wilmink, R., and Croughs, W.: Aldosterone and cortisol secretion rates in infants and children with congenital adrenal hyperplasia suggesting different 21-hydroxylation defects in salt-losers and non salt-losers. Acta Endocrinol., *48:* 587, 1965.
12. Dignam, W. J., Pion, R. J., Lamb, E. J., and Simmer, H. H.: Plasma androgens in women. II. Patients with polycystic ovaries and hirsutism. Acta Endocrinol., *45:* 254, 1964.
13. Dingemanse, E., and Hius, In't Veld, L. G.: Origin of the androsterone in the urine of women. Acta Endocrinol., *7:* 71, 1951.

14. Eberlein, W. R., and Bongiovanni, A. M.: Defective steroidal biogenesis in congenital adrenal hyperplasia. Pediatrics, *21:* 661, 1958.
15. Finkelstein, M., Forchielli, E., and Dorfman, R. I.: Estimation of testosterone in human plasma. J. Clin. Endocrinol., *21:* 98, 1961.
16. Forchielli, E., Sarcini, G., Nightingale, M. S., Brust, N., Dorfman, R. I., Perloff, W. H., and Jacobson, G.: Testosterone in human plasma. Ann. Biochem., *5:* 416, 1963.
17. French, F. S., Baggett, B., Van Wyk, J. J., Talbert, L. M., Hubbart, W. R., Johnston, F. R., Weaver, R. P., Forchielli, E., Rao, G. S., and Sarda, I. R.: Testicular feminization: clinical, morphological and biochemical studies. J. Clin. Endocrinol., *25:* 661, 1965.
18. Gallagher, T. F., Kappas, A., Hellman, L., Lipsett, M. B., Pearson, O. H., and West, C. D.: Adrenocortical hyperfunction in idiopathic hirsutism and the Stein-Leventhal syndrome. J. Clin. Invest., *37:* 794, 1958.
19. Gemzell, C. A., Diczfalusy, E., and Tillinger, K. G.: Clinical effect of human pituitary follicle-stimulating hormone (FSH). J. Clin. Endocrinol., *18:* 1333, 1958.
20. Gemzell, C. A., Tillinger, K., and Westman, A.: Hirsutism: a clinical study of ovarian pathology and the urinary excretion of 17-ketosteroids. Acta Endocrinol. (Kbh), *30:* 387, 1959.
21. Goldzieher, J. W., and Axelrod, L. R.: Adrenal and ovarian steroid genesis in the sclerocystic ovary syndrome. Acta Endocrinol. (Kbh) Supp., *51:* 617, 1960.
22. Goldzieher, J. W., and Axelrod, L. R.: The polycystic ovary. II. Urinary steroid excretion. J. Clin. Endocrinol., *22:* 425, 1962.
23. Greenblatt, R. B.: Cortisone in treatment of hirsute women. Am. J. Obst. & Gynec., *66:* 700, 1953.
24. Greenblatt, R. B.: Clinical aspects of sexual abnormalities in man. Recent Progr. in Hormone Res., *14:* 335, 1958.
25. Greenblatt, R. B., Dominguez, H., Mahesh, V. B., and Demos, R.: Gonadal dysgenesis intersex with XO-XY mosaicism. J.A.M.A., *188:* 221, 1964.
26. Herrmann, W., Buckner, F., and Morris, J. M.: The problem of "mild" adrenal hyperplasia. Fertil. & Steril., *11:* 74, 1960.
27. Hudson, B., Coghlan, J., Dulmanis, A., Wintour, M., and Ekkel, I.: The estimation of testosterone in biological fluids. 1. Testosterone in plasma. Australian J. Exper. Biol. & M. Sc., *41:* 235, 1963.
28. Jailer, J. W.: Virilism. Bull. New York Acad. Med., *29:* 377, 1953.
29. Jayle, M. F., Scholler, R., Mauvais-Jarvis, P., and Metay, S.: Excretion of steroids in women with pilary virilism associated with

disorders of the menstrual cycle. Acta Endocrinol. (Kbh), *36:* 375, 1961.
30. Keetall, W. C., Bradbury, J. T., and Stoddard, F. J.: Observations on the polycystic ovary syndrome. Am. J. Obst. & Gynec., *73:* 954, 1957.
31. Korenman, S. G., and Lipsett, M. B.: Direct peripheral conversion of dehydroepiandrosterone to testosterone glucuronoside. Steroids, *5:* 509, 1965.
32. Lipsett, M. B., and Riter, B.: Urinary ketosteroids and pregnanetriol in hirsutism. J. Clin. Endocrinol., *20:* 180, 1960.
33. MacDonald, P., Vande Wiele, R. L., and Lieberman, S.: Precursors of the urinary 11-desoxy-17-ketosteroids of ovarian origin. Am. J. Obst. and Gynec., *86:* 1, 1963.
34. Mahesh, V. B., and Greenblatt, R. B.: The in vivo conversion of dehydroepiandrosterone and androstenedione to testosterone in the human. Acta Endocrinol., *41:* 400, 1962.
35. Mahesh, V. B., and Greenblatt, R. B.: Urinary steroid excretion patterns in hirsutism. II. Effect of ovarian stimulation with human pituitary FSH on urinary 17-ketosteroids. J. Clin. Endocrinol., *24:* 1293, 1964.
36. Mahesh, V. B., and Greenblatt, R. B.: Isolation of dehydroepiandrosterone and 17α-hydroxy-Δ5-pregnenalone from the polycystic ovaries of the Stein-Leventhal syndrome. J. Clin. Endocrinol., *22:* 441, 1962.
37. Mahesh, V. B., and Greenblatt, R. B.: Physiology and pathogenesis of the Stein-Leventhal syndrome. Nature, *191:* 888, 1961.
38. Mahesh, V. B., and Greenblatt, R. B.: Proceedings of the 6th Pan American Congress of Endocrinology, International Congress Series #99 of the 6th Annual Proceedings of the Pan American Congress of Endocrinology, 1965.
39. Mahesh, V. B., and Greenblatt, R. B.: Steroid secretions of the normal and polycystic ovary. Recent Progr. Hormone Res., *20:* 341, 1964.
40. Mahesh, V. B., Greenblatt, R. B., Aydar, C. K., and Roy, S.: Secretion of androgen by the polycystic ovary and its significance. Fertil. & Steril., *13:* 513, 1962.
41. Mahesh, V. B., Greenblatt, R. B., Aydar, C. K., Roy, S., Puebla, R. A., and Ellegood, J. O.: Urinary steroid excretion patterns in hirsutism. I. Use of adrenal and ovarian suppression tests in the study of hirsutism. J. Clin. Endocrinol., *24:* 1283, 1964.
42. Morris, J. M., and Mahesh, V. B.: Further observations on the syndrome, "testicular feminization." Am. J. Obst. & Gynec., *87:* 731, 1963.

43. Netter, A., Jayle, M. F., Musset, R., Lambert, A., and Mauvais-Jarvis, P.: Dynamic tests in Stein-Leventhal syndrome. Ann. Endocrinol. (Paris), *21:* 590, 1960.
44. Perloff, W. H.: Hirsutism—manifestations of juvenile hypothyroidism. J.A.M.A., *157:* 651, 1955.
45. Perloff, W. H., Channick, B. J., Suplick, B., and Carrington, E. R.: Clinical management of idiopathic hirsutism (adrenal virilism). J.A.M.A., *167*,2041, 1958.
46. Pesonen, S., Timonen, S., and Mikkonen, R.: Symptoms and etiology of the Stein-Leventhal syndrome. Acta Endocrinol. (Kbh), *30:* 405, 1959.
47. Riondel, A., Tait, J. F., Gut, M., Tait, S. A. S., Joachim, E., and Little, B.: Estimation of testosterone in human peripheral blood using S35-thiosemicarbazide. J. Clin. Endocrinol., *23:* 620, 1963.
48. Shepard, T. H., and Clausen, S. W.: Case of adrenogenital syndrome with hypertension treated with cortisone. Pediatrics, *8:* 805, 1951.
49. Southren, A. L., Ross, H., Sharma, D. C., Gordon, G., Weingold, A. B., and Dorfman, R. I.: Plasma concentration and biosynthesis of testosterone in the syndrome of feminizing testes. J. Clin. Endocrinol., *25:* 518, 1965.
50. Stein, I. F., and Leventhal, M. L.: Amenorrhea associated with bilateral polycystic ovaries. Am. J. Obst. & Gynec., *29:* 181, 1935.
51. Tait, J. F., and Horton, R.: Some theoretical considerations on the significance in the discrepancy in urinary and blood production rate estimates of steroid hormones particularly in those of testosterone in young women. Steroids, *4:* 365, 1964.
52. Turner, H., Greenblatt, R. B., and Dominguez, H.: Syndrome of gonadal dysgenesis and abdominal testis with an XO/XY chromosome mosaicism. J. Clin. Endocrinol., *23:* 709, 1963.
53. Vande Wiele, R., MacDonald, P. C., Gurpide, E., and Lieberman, S.: Studies on the secretion and interconversion of the androgens. Recent Progr. Hormone Res., *19:* 275, 1963.
54. Wilkins, L., Lewis, R. A., Klein, R., and Rosemberg, E.: Suppression of androgen secretion by cortisone in case of congenital adrenal hyperplasia. Bull. Johns Hopkins Hosp., *86:* 249, 1950.
55. Wilkins, L., Lewis, R. A., Klein, R., Gardner, L. I., Crigler, J. F., Rosenberg, E., and Migeon, C. J.: Treatment of congenital adrenal hyperplasia with cortisone. J. Clin. Endocrinol., *11:* 1, 1951.
56. Zourlas, P. A., and Jones, H. W.: Clinical, histologic, and cytogenetic findings in male hermaphroditism. 3. Male hermaphrodites with asymmetrical gonadal differentiation (mixed gonadal dysgenesis). Obst. & Gynec., *26:* 48, 1965.

8

Vaginitis

Alexander M. Burnett, M.D.

This paper reviews the gynecological experience over a 30-month period in the adolescent clinic of the Children's Hospital in Washington, D.C.

In 1960, Dr. Heald and Dr. Sturgis reviewed their experience over a 5-year period at Children's Hospital in Boston.[2] In their article they state that while careful examination of the external genitalia for vaginal discharge and abnormalities was carried out in all cases, vaginal examination was not routinely performed but when deemed necessary was done under general anesthesia. Allen[1] has stated that, if girls are gradually conditioned to a vaginal examination prior to the menarche, it will be accepted as part of the routine examination during adolescence.

Because of the high rate of coitus found among the patients seen by us in the adolescent clinic, the inability to carry out a satisfactory pelvic examination has been the exception rather than the rule. In fact, the majority of problems encountered have been similar to those which one would expect in a more adult population. Our observations point out that there are many social as well as medical problems in this area.

A high percentage of our patients had overt evidence of sexual exposure as is apparent from the diagnostic classification in Table 8.1. It was found that 15 were pregnant, and 11 showed evidence of pelvic inflammatory disease.

TABLE 8.1
Diagnostic Classification

Vaginitis and vulvitis	25
Pregnancy or suspected pregnancy	15
Pelvic infection	12
Congenital abnormalities	5
Dysmenorrhea	8
Metropathia hemorrhagica	10

TABLE 8.2
Age Distribution of Patients

Age	No. of Patients
yrs.	
18	1
17	1
16	10
15	4
14	5
13	3
12	1

Our attention currently is directed to the adolescent who complains of vaginal discharge. Of the total number of girls 25, or one-third, were referred for this complaint. Of the 25, 23 girls were 16 years old or younger (Table 8.2).

Of this group, 21 admitted to previous sexual contact and 20 of them could be examined pelvically (Table 8.3). Thus, out of a total of 75 girls, 47 admitted to previous sexual contact.

Vaginal discharge for which a patient will seek medical attention can vary from the profuse, frothy, foul smelling, and pruritic variety associated with the classical case of Trichomonas vaginitis to the small amount of clear mucoid, whitish discharge which is asymptomatic and which is physiologically found prior to the onset of menstruation and often at ovulation. No therapy was advised in those cases in which no overt evidence of vulvitis or clinical vaginitis was found, in which the vagina and cervix were found to be clean by inspection at least with the small Pederson speculum, and in which no pathological organisms were grown on culture.

Table 8.4 shows the results of vaginal cultures. While the ma-

TABLE 8.3
History of Coitus and Pelvic Examination

	Yes	No
Coitus	21	4
Pelvic examination	20	5

TABLE 8.4
Results of Vaginal Cultures

Staphylococcus albus	10
Diphtheroids	9
Trichomonas	9
Candida	7
E. coli	4
Staphylococcus aureus	1
B hemolytic streptococcus	1
Aerobacter	1
Proteus mirabilis	1

jority of the organisms were those normally found in the vagina, i.e., *Staphylococcus albus* and diphtheroids, there was a reasonably high incidence of *Trichomonas vaginalis* and *Monilia albicans*.

In this series congenital erosion or eversion of the cervix was not thought to be the sole cause of discharge in any of the cases.

VAGINAL INFECTIONS

1. Trichomonas vaginalis

This protozoan flagellate may be in the vagina without producing symptoms. Typically, it leads to an acute vaginitis with a frothy, yellow-green discharge. There is often an associated vulvitis. On examination of the vagina, one frequently sees small hemorrhagic areas of inflammation known as "strawberry vaginitis." The diagnosis is confirmed by finding in a wet smear, prepared by adding one drop of warm isotonic saline to one drop of the discharge, the typical organism which is about twice the size of a leukocyte, and has an undulating membrane and usually multiple flagella.

Treatment usually consists of cleansing douches, often with vinegar, in an attempt to restore the normal pH of the vagina, coupled with a trichomonacidal agent. Because this has been a difficult organism to eradicate, there have been many therapeutic agents recommended.

Since many have considered this organism to be venereal in the sense that its perpetuation can be effected by an asymptomatically infected male partner, an orally efficacious remedy has been sought for both male and female. Over the last several years, excellent results have been reported with the use of metronidazole or Flagyl.* This may be given as a combined course of oral and vaginal therapy: oral tablets 250 mg. b.i.d. and vaginal suppository 500 mg. once daily. We have used this drug in 6 patients with good to excellent results and no recurrence of acute disease.

2. *Candida albicans*

This yeast-like organism may cause severe symptoms, especially those of pruritus and burning. Frequently, vaginitis may be associated with vulvitis and intertrigonitis. The discharge is typically white, curdy, and often adherent to the vaginal wall. It may be diagnosed by finding the fiber-like mycelia and spores of candida on a wet smear to which one drop of 10 per cent potassium hydroxide has been added, or by streaking of Nickerson's medium at room temperature. The growth of black colonies 1 to 2 mm. in diameter are diagnostic. It should be pointed out that Candida albicans is commonly associated with three entities: (a) the use of broad spectrum antibiotics, (b) pregnancy, and (c) diabetes mellitus. In our series of cases 1 patient was pregnant and 2 had diabetes mellitus.

3. *Nonspecific vaginitis*

This is commonly diagnosed when an excessive amount of discharge coupled with symptoms of vaginitis occur. At Georgetown University we have cultured Hemophilus vaginalis frequently together with other organisms from this type of vaginitis. However, there is commonly no uniformity of growth on culture.

Vinegar douches coupled with AVC* or Sultrin* cream are commonly used as therapy for this condition. The creams mentioned are combinations of sulfanilamide with various antifungal and antiparasitic components which amounts to nonspecific therapy for nonspecific disease.

* ®

4. Neisseria gonorrhoeae

The leukorrhea observed with pelvic inflammatory disease secondary to gonococcal infections is usually mucopurulent in character and profuse in amount. It normally responds effectively to the treatment of the causative organism with penicillin or other effective antibiotic drugs. Symptomatic relief may be afforded by the use of cleansing warm water douches.

Of the 11 patients referred to the adolescent clinic with tentative diagnosis of pelvic inflammatory disease, in only 1 were gram negative intracellular diplococci seen. In no instance was Neisseria gonorrhoeae grown on culture. Nearly all of these patients were seen in the emergency room and therapy had been initiated before we saw them.

It appears from our results that a very real sociological problem exists which has been known to members of our specialty dealing with adolescent patients for years. Adolescents of low socioeconomic groups in large American cities establish sexual relationships at a very young age which leads to numerous problems in the realm of medicine.

REFERENCES

1. Allen, E. D.: Examination of the genital organs in the prepubescent and in the adolescent girl. Pediat. Clin. North America, 5: 19, 1958.
2. Heald, F. P., and Sturgis, S. H.: Adolescent gynecology—a 5-year study. Pediatrics, 25: 669, 1960.

9

Public Health Aspects of Venereal Disease

William J. Dougherty, M.D.

A brief historical review of syphilis and gonorrhea in the United States is necessary for an appraisal of the public health aspects of venereal disease control as currently practiced.

In 1932 Parran said: "Syphilis can never be controlled while more than one-half of the cases are not recognized for more than one year after onset." [11]

In 1936 Parran reported upon the recommendations of a national conference on veneral disease control as follows: Find, report and interview for sex contacts every early case of syphilis. Treat every case. Align health agencies and private physicians in a united front. Case finding was the major weapon in the control of syphilis.

For a period of approximately 15 years, prior to 1936, the incidence rate of syphilis in all stages varied between 150 and 200 cases per 100,000 population.

Figure 9.1 indicates that a marked increase in incidence occurred in 1936. In response to Surgeon General Parran's efforts, the index of suspicion for syphilis was markedly increased, and prenatal, premarital, and hospital admission serological screening programs came into being.

The screening of over 13 million candidates for the Armed Forces by selective service increased the incidence of reported syphilis during the war years.

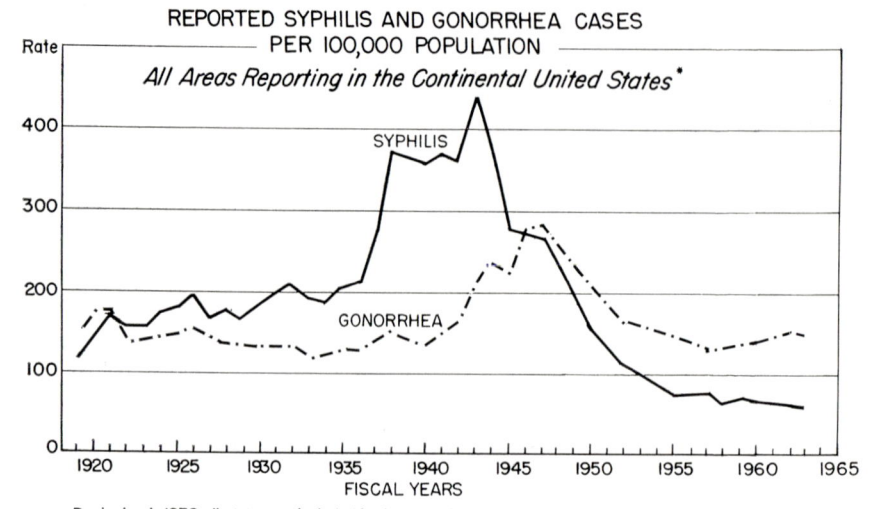

REPORTED SYPHILIS AND GONORRHEA CASES PER 100,000 POPULATION
All Areas Reporting in the Continental United States*

* Beginning in 1939 all states are included in the reporting area.
(Military cases included 1919-1940, excluded thereafter)

FIG. 9.1

The decline following the year 1945 may be associated with the massive case finding effort in the preceding 10 years, and the extensive venereal disease control program carried on during the war. These efforts may have succeeded in drying up the reservoir of infectious syphilis. The advent of penicillin, which rapidly controlled the infectious stage of syphilis, may have accelerated the decline also. Since 1952 the over-all rate for syphilis in the United States has been less than 100 cases per 100,000 a year.

The rate at which gonorrhea was reported remained almost stable for a period of 20 years. Under the impact of the venereal disease control program during World War II, the rate nearly doubled. As the control program declined, so did the reporting of gonorrhea until, in 1955, the reporting level approximated that of 1920 to 1940.

Figure 9.2, prepared from New Jersey data, indicates that for a period of 20 years there was a slow relatively stable decline in the numbers of cases of syphilis in all stages.

The discrepancy between the numbers of cases of early latent syphilis and primary-secondary syphilis from 1948 to 1955 is remarkable. Each case of early latent syphilis reported in that pe-

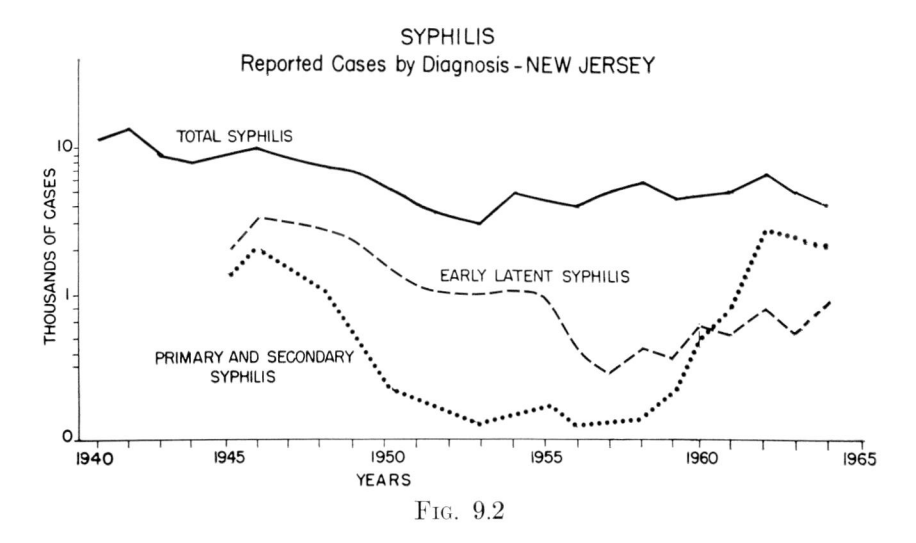

SYPHILIS
Reported Cases by Diagnosis - NEW JERSEY

FIG. 9.2

riod represents a case of syphilis which had been undiscovered in its primary or secondary stage. The reasons for this discrepancy are not clear but may include unreported and inadequately treated primary-secondary syphilis, or syphilis masked by the widespread use of penicillin in the treatment of many other diseases, or the lack of epidemiological investigation to determine the sources and spread of primary-secondary syphilis. In any event, it appears that constant transmission of syphilis occurred at a rate which did not justify the enthusiasm which accompanied the decline in the primary-secondary syphilis curve.

The numbers of cases of primary-secondary, early latent, and total syphilis and gonorrhea reported to the Public Health Service in 4 recent years are presented in Table 9.1. The 22,733 cases of primary-secondary syphilis reported in 1964 approach 4 times the number reported at the low point in 1957. "This is the highest reported incidence level since 1950." [12]

The ratio of primary-secondary syphilis to early latent syphilis has been interpreted as an index of primary-secondary syphilis case finding. When the number of infectious cases exceeds the number of early latent cases, spread of the disease is inhibited through early treatment. When early latent cases exceed the number of infectious cases, spread of the disease is not inhibited

TABLE 9.1

Reported Syphilis and Gonorrhea in the United States

Year	Syphilis			Gonorrhea
	Primary-secondary	Early latent	Total	
1957	6251	19,046	130,552	216,476
1962	20,084	19,924	124,188	260,468
1963	22,045	18,683	128,450	270,076
1964	22,733	18,106	118,268	291,598

since the majority of cases progress completely through the infectious stage before they are detected. In 1957 there were 6251 cases of primary-secondary syphilis compared to 19,046 cases of early latent syphilis. It is apparent that the case finding was low and spread of disease was not inhibited. In 1964 the relationship was modified to a point where 22,733 cases of primary-secondary syphilis were being reported compared to 18,106 cases of early latent syphilis.

In 1962 there were 19,924 cases of early latent syphilis reported compared to 18,106 in 1964. The decrease in early latent cases in spite of an increase in infectious cases indicates to some degree that a higher proportion of infected persons were found in the primary and secondary stage, thus preventing progression and transmission of the disease.

There is a noticeable trend in the decline of the total cases of syphilis in all stages reported to the Public Health Service. This drop reflects a continuing decline in the numbers of cases of late and late latent syphilis which have decreased almost every year since 1943 when 251,958 cases were reported.[12] Nevertheless, while the numbers of old untreated cases are diminishing, there remains a considerable reservoir of disease and disability to be discovered and controlled.

The numbers of cases of gonorrhea have increased steadily each year since 1957 at a slightly faster rate than the population has grown. The 291,598 cases reported in 1964 make gonorrhea one of the most frequently reported of the nationally notifiable diseases.[14]

There is some evidence that the increase in reported gonorrhea cases may represent better reporting of the disease rather than an actual upturn in incidence. The evidence supporting this indication is a sharp upturn in the reporting of gonorrhea cases by private physicians.[2]

There were 3728 cases of congenital syphilis reported in 1964.[13] It is estimated that only 347 cases of congenital syphilis were among infants less than 1 year of age. The bulk of congenital cases being reported in the United States today is among adults who were born with syphilis years ago. There can be no complacency, for high rates of infectious syphilis exist among persons in the childbearing age. The risk of congenital syphilis is striking; a recent study in 27 states indicates that, among 995,000 persons receiving a premarital blood test, there were 12,250 persons who were serologically positive for syphilis, a rate of 1.2 per cent.[3]

It is disturbing that 1 person out of 81 marriage applicants was found to be serologically positive for syphilis.

In the same study, 23 states reported that 962,000 prenatal tests were given during the year; 9724 were positive, a rate of 1 per cent. This yield of prenatal positives is disturbing. One out of every 100 prospective mothers tested was suspected of having syphilis.

In this study, most of the cities and states indicated that their premarital blood testing approached 100 per cent completeness. Prenatal blood testing was reported as less complete, and many states and cities qualified their opinions as to the completeness by stating that prenatal testing was not done where the woman did not receive prenatal care. The proportion of such cases varies according to social and economic factors present in different areas.

Data obtained in a study of congenital syphilis conducted in New Jersey between January and December 1963 are presented in Tables 9.2 and 9.3. This study involved investigation of 83 infants, 20 of whom came to attention because of a report of congenital syphilis received by the State Department of Health; 63 infants were called to attention because of laboratory reports suggestive of syphilis. In this investigation, a Public Health nurse worked directly with the physicians who reported the cases or the pediatric clinics to which the cases were referred as the result of a reactive serological test for syphilis.

In all, 16 infants were discovered who could be diagnosed truly as having congenital syphilis. Another 15 infants were found on

TABLE 9.2

Congenital Syphilis in New Jersey—January 1 to December 31, 1963

Source of Information	No. of Infants	Investigation Complete	Incomplete
Total	95	83	12
Disease reports	20	20	0
Serology reports	75	63	12

TABLE 9.3

Congenital Syphilis in New Jersey—January 1 to December 31, 1963

Source of Information	Number	Completed Investigations in Infants – Infected	Epidemiological treatment	No treatment, not infected
Total	83	16	15	52
Disease reports	20	4	4	12
Serology reports	63	12	11	40

investigation to have been treated shortly after birth, and thus a clear-cut clinical diagnosis could not be established.

Note that 12 of the infants originally reported as having disease were found on careful follow-up examinations to be free of infection.

A more important observation from this study, however, is the fact that over 45 per cent of the mothers of these infants had received no prenatal care prior to delivery. Another group appeared for prenatal care in the last trimester only. It is sufficient to say that the ingredients are present for an outbreak of congenital syphilis in some areas among low income groups.

There is continued concern about the spread of syphilis between persons of the same sex. Table 9.4 demonstrates the ratio of male to female syphilis over a period of several years. This table alone is not conclusive evidence of homosexuality, but it is supported by the results of interviewing and investigating cases of syphilis. Table 9.5 indicates the number of male contacts that were found in a chain of homosexual syphilis several years ago.

Recently, 31 states reported that 1621 males with infectious syphilis named male contacts, and 11 states reported that 57 females with infectious syphilis named female contacts.[4] In this

TABLE 9.4

Ratio of Male to Female Cases of Primary-Secondary Syphilis in United States—1959-1963

Year	White	Nonwhite	Total
	ratio M/F		
1959	4.53	1.55	2.19
1960	5.14	1.51	2.26
1961	4.53	1.58	2.15
1962	4.22	1.45	1.92
1963	3.75	1.49	1.86

TABLE 9.5

Early Syphilis Epidemiological Chain in Homosexual Males—New Jersey, 1960

Classification	No. of Persons
Contacts	25
Suspects	133
Total	158

study, cities reported a decline in males with infectious syphilis naming male sex partners. This trend was offset by the male homosexual trend reported by states.

There are several possible explanations for this apparent contradiction. Some city health departments may be so alert to the problem that intensive epidemiology among the homosexual group has resulted in a decrease in the number of syphilis infections transmitted from male to male.

In regard to syphilis and homosexuality among female patients, it must be noted that the numbers are small and that female transmission is a rare occurrence, if indeed it occurs at all. Reinterviews on female patients usually produce at least one male contact who may be involved in the chain of infection. On the other hand, the number of male homosexuals transmitting syphilis represents a sizable problem in syphilis control.

Thus far, we have spoken of reported cases of syphilis and gonorrhea. It is important that we estimate the degree to which the diseases are underreported.

In 1962 the American Social Health Association, through the cooperation of the American Medical Association, the American Osteopathic Association, and the National Medical Association conducted a mail survey of all physicians in general practice and in medical specialties in the United States.[9] The survey questionnaire was a three-question form, requesting the number of new cases of primary-secondary syphilis, of other stages of syphilis, and of gonorrhea treated in a three-month period from April 1 to June 30, 1962. Of the 184,500 physicians contacted, a total of 131,251 responded, a rate of 71 per cent. Of these respondents, 34 per cent indicated that they had treated some form of venereal disease during the three-month period. The percentage of physicians treating venereal disease was greatest among the general practitioner group, 57 per cent, while only 21 per cent of the specialists reported having patients with venereal disease.

The physicians responding to the questionnaire indicated that they had treated 19,930 patients with infectious syphilis but only 1576 cases had been reported to the state health departments during the same three-month period. They treated 34,069 patients with other stages of syphilis, and 12,785 of these were reported. Of the 156,515 cases of gonorrhea treated, only 16,907 were reported to the health departments. These figures indicate that only 11.3 per cent of the cases of infectious syphilis, 37.5 per cent of cases of other syphilis, and 10.8 per cent of the cases of gonorrhea treated by private physicians during the three-month survey period were reported to the health departments.

Replies to the survey questionnaire indicated that private physicians were treating by conservative estimate 76 per cent of the venereal disease cases in the United States. Thus, less than one-fourth of the venereal disease cases are being treated in public health clinics and institutions where adequate follow-up procedures concerning sexual contacts are in operation.

Each case of infectious syphilis that is not identified, reported, and processed epidemiologically does four things to the community: it contributes to the spread of disease; it increases the existing infectious syphilis reservoir; it eventually results in a higher attack rate in the population; and it positively prevents any possibility for the control of syphilis.

Without going into the mathematics of the estimate, using the data provided by the survey and knowledge concerning the reporting of clinic patients, it is estimated that a total of about 100,000 to 140,000 cases of infectious syphilis are being identified and treated annually. In a similar fashion, it is estimated that Americans are contracting gonorrhea at a rate exceeding 85 thousand cases a month or more than a million per year.[1] The resurgence of venereal diseases is not limited to the North American continent. The World Health Organization estimates that 60 million new cases of gonorrhea occur annually throughout the world.

We must answer the question of where venereal diseases are occurring. Figure 9.3 indicates those areas of the United States in which infectious syphilis is an important problem.

In a recent study by the American Social Health Association, evidence was obtained which indicates that 112 cities, whose aggregate population represents 30.7 per cent of the total population of the United States, reported 57 per cent of all infectious syphilis and 64.5 per cent of all gonorrhea.[2]

A fact that should be faced and faced without flinching is that 30 cities with less than one-fifth of our population are harboring syphilis epidemics at this very moment, in many cases not only virtually ignored but often vigorously denied.[6] Table 9.6 provides a vivid example of a city in the throes of an epidemic for 2 years.

The high proportion of infectious venereal disease among teenagers and young adults has been receiving increasing attention in this country. The national statistics of primary-secondary syphilis by age are available for the calendar year 1963.[5] They are worthy of study. In that year 40 cases of primary-secondary syphilis were reported in the age group 0 to 9 years, 233 cases in the age group 10 to 14 years, 3438 cases in the 15 to 19 year age group, and 6332 cases in the 20 to 24 age group. Infectious syphilis patients under 25 years of age numbered 10,043, accounting for 44.9 per cent of the total infectious syphilis morbidity reporting during the year.

Table 9.7 presents the trend of incidence of primary-secondary syphilis by age in New Jersey. Note that in 1958 in the 15 to 19 age group, there were 7 cases per 100,000, and by 1963 the rate had increased to 38.6. Note also the increase in the age group 20 to 24 years, from 13.0 per 100,000 in 1958 to 107.3 per 100,000 in 1963.

Nationally in 1963, 157,098 cases of gonorrhea were reported in the age group under 25 or 56.3 per cent of all reported gonorrhea. It is of interest that the 98,541 cases in the age group 20 to 24

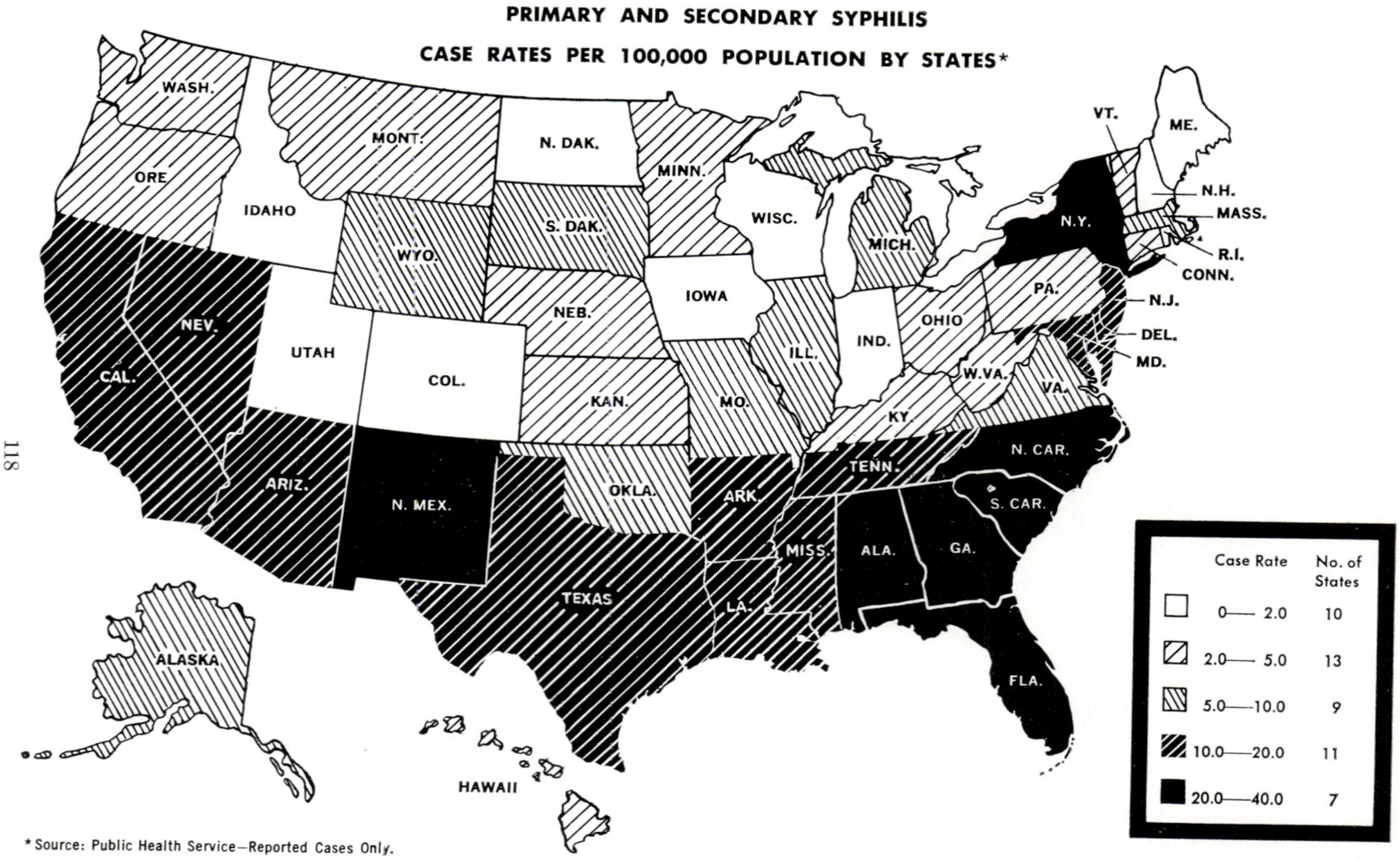
PRIMARY AND SECONDARY SYPHILIS
CASE RATES PER 100,000 POPULATION BY STATES*
WASH.
ORE
IDAHO
MONT.
WYO.
N. DAK.
S. DAK.
NEB.
MINN.
WISC.
IOWA
MICH.
ILL.
IND.
OHIO
PA.
N.Y.
VT.
ME.
N.H.
MASS.
R.I.
CONN.
N.J.
DEL.
MD.
W.VA.
VA.
KY.
MO.
KAN.
COL.
UTAH
NEV.
CAL.
ARIZ.
N. MEX.
OKLA.
TEXAS
ARK.
LA.
MISS.
TENN.
ALA.
GA.
N. CAR.
S. CAR.
FLA.
ALASKA
HAWAII
Case Rate
No. of States
0—2.0 10
2.0—5.0 13
5.0—10.0 9
10.0—20.0 11
20.0—40.0 7

* Source: Public Health Service—Reported Cases Only.

FIG. 9.3

TABLE 9.6
Reported Early Syphilis Case Rate per 100,000 Population in Newark City

Year	Syphilis	
	Primary-secondary	Early latent
1957	8.0	27.3
1960	76.0	69.1
1963	103.0	74.1

TABLE 9.7
Primary–Secondary Syphilis Rates per 100,000—New Jersey, 1958–1963

Age	1958	1962	1963
Under 1			1.5
1–4		0.4	
5–14	0.6	2.6	0.8
15–19	7.1	39.1	38.6
20–24	13.5	106.4	107.3
25–44	5.0	35.3	31.3
45 and over	0.6	3.3	3.1

years is the highest number of cases ever reported in this age group since age data have been collected.[3]

Figure 9.4 shows the areas of the country in which infectious venereal disease among teenagers constitutes a severe public health problem. This figure illustrates dramatically the reasons for concern about venereal infection in young people. Thus, stress has been placed upon the need for an informational, educational program which is directed specifically at the younger age groups. Special emphasis has been placed upon venereal disease education in the schools, as the majority of the teenagers are in schools and can be reached before they have completed school and have become widely dispersed. The difficulty of reaching the 20 to 24 year age group in which infection is the most prevalent makes it mandatory that information and education about venereal disease be given to teenagers who will soon join the older group.

We have seen the extent to which infectious venereal disease has spread in this country. The American Medical Association meeting in San Francisco last June, 1964, adopted the following resolution:

"Resolved that the House of Delegates take official cognizance

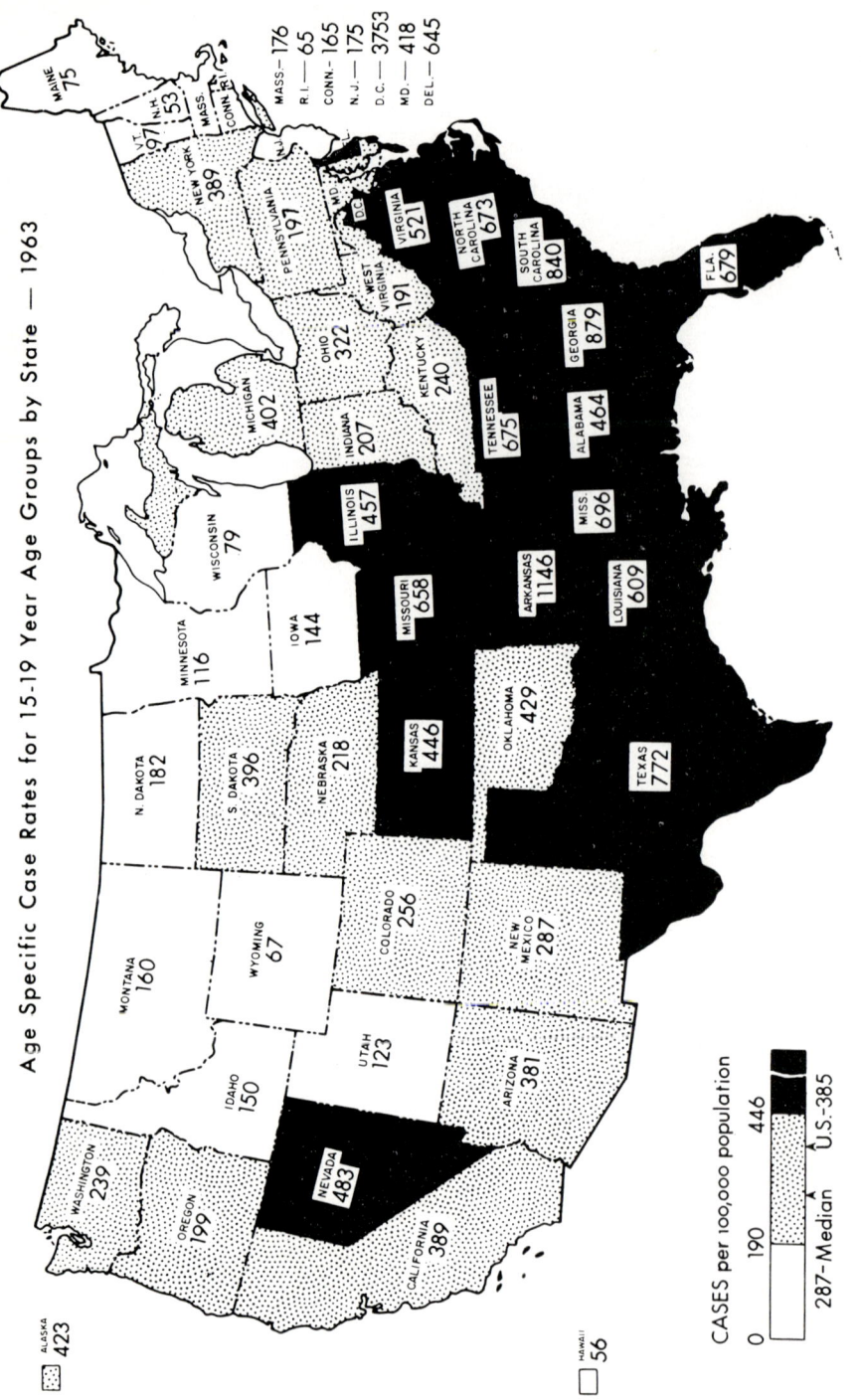

FIG. 9.4

of the resurgence of syphilis and gonorrhea to the proportions of a national health problem; that it initiate... a comprehensive inquiry of the positive factors of this sharp increase in disease for which a simple cure is now available; that it take leadership in educational and research measures designed to control and eliminate syphilis; and that it provide guidance to private physicians in the epidemiology of the venereal diseases and their social implications." [7]

We have seen medical leadership combat another disease. In city after city, local medical societies in rapid order have taken hold of the Salk and Sabin vaccines and in all practicality have effected the eradication of polio. There is no reason why they cannot do the same for syphilis. The tools of eradication are indeed at hand. The only thing required is the decision to put them to work and that decision is taking shape in many quarters.

Recently, "the Public Health Committee of the New York Academy of Medicine granted as unacceptable the failure of any physician to report morbidity or to grant permission to have syphilis patients interviewed for contacts. It called morbidity reporting and the employment of public health epidemiologic assistance the physician's duty and responsibility and it denied that such action infringes on the rights of patients or constitutes a breach of professional privilege. If the private physician has on tap a highly intelligent well-trained professional assistant, perfectly capable of rendering efficient confidential service to him and to his patient, and one who can assist materially in the fulfillment of his professional obligations, who could doubt that he would long refrain from making use of such an assistant." [8]

The use of the public health epidemiologist not only will bring to the physician's doorstep the manifest cases of infectious syphilis. Also through the efforts of the epidemiologist, the physician will discover a group of patients who, from the standpoint of eradication, are perhaps even more important, that is the select group of contacts who while they lack lesions, while their blood is still sero-negative, include in their midst a full 10 per cent of their number who are incubating syphilis. This is a very important group because recent studies show that for every 100 asymptomatically sero-negative contacts to infectious syphilis not treated prophylactically, 10 will develop infectious lesions and these 10 will pass their infections to 5 additional persons before they can be diagnosed.[10]

After 10 years of deemphasis on syphilology, it is an understandably difficult task to persuade a busy practitioner to stay constantly on the alert for new infections and to get excited over a single case which may be the only one he sees in a year. Yet, if we fail to persuade him to do exactly this, we run the risk of undetected infectious syphilis, and thus the source of infection is not traced or treated.

It is not unreasonable to expect the physician to initiate diagnostic tests on two categories of patients—those appearing in his office with lesions suggestive of syphilis and those appearing without lesions but mentioning or suggesting the possibility of exposure. Modern blood testing procedures are not difficult or expensive, and dark field examination of lesions is becoming more practicable. Where there are open lesions and the physician does not have dark field equipment, expert dark field services are now available on call from many if not all health departments.

The State of New Jersey maintains a 24-hour answering service. A physician may call and request dark field services from the State Health Department. An epidemiologist is assigned to serve the physician within an hour or two. If immediate service is impossible or inconvenient, the physician may arrange with his patient to return to his office for an appointment within 24 hours. At that time the epidemiologist will be in the office prepared to render service. The important aspect of this service is that the epidemiologist who prepares the dark field examination is in contact with the patient at the moment of diagnosis and is able to interview him for sex contacts at a most opportune time. With every hour that passes after adequate treatment, the patient's interest not only in his own disease but also in the people with whom he may have been associated becomes less and less.

The first step in the epidemiological investigation of syphilis is, of course, the diagnosis. We cannot overstress the importance of doing a complete physical examination—dermal, oral, anal, and genital. We are quite certain that we will miss syphilis unless each person is completely examined, all orifices and the entire body surface. The second element of the investigation is case reporting. There is no investigation if the case is not reported to the health department. The epidemiological interview is the third step. In this interview, a trained epidemiologist determines the extent of the patient's sexual activity and the numbers of contacts that the patient has had within 6 months of the onset of symptoms. The investigator must obtain adequate identifying information so that contacts and suspects can be located and brought to treatment. Epidemiologists have followed many persons in many parts of the world by means of the communication chain which now exists between the states and between the United States and other nations. The fourth step includes a re-interviewing of patients to amplify information that was incomplete and to improve initial locating information that proved to be inadequate.

The epidemiological interview begins with a discussion between the epidemiologist and the physician, in which the epidemiologist obtains from the physician information which will assist in interviewing the patient. Many epidemiologists have developed excellent working relationships with physicians over a period of years. To assist in establishing this rapport, epidemiologists are assigned to visit physicians in their offices to discuss the incidence of syphilis in the state and to explain the services made available to the physician by the state department of health and the assistance which the epidemiologist can render to the physician and to his patients. Once this rapport is established, we find that the physicians begin to call the epidemiologist when they have patients for whom they need service.

The next step involves locating the patient. It is important that adequate identifying information be given by the physician in order that the patient can be found for interview. There is still a sense of shame associated with contracting a venereal disease. Many people fail to give their right names, their right addresses and may seek physician services in communities where they are not known. The venereal disease patient seeks anonymity. Essentially, we want to avoid wasting time on investigations that are fruitless.

Once the epidemiologist is in contact with the patient, the interview is held. At this point the epidemiologist puts into practice his skill as an interviewer. In the interview, he attempts to develop a general history of the patients sexual experience. Several of his questions are as follows: When did you first become aware of your sex? When did you first become aware of the other sex? When did you first engage in sex play? At what point in life did you have your first sexual experience? When did you have your last experience? The whole purpose of the interview is to establish a series of limits within which the patient's exposure to infectious syphilis can be determined. Finally, more specific questions are raised: How frequently have you had sexual intercourse in the last 6 months? With whom have you had sexual intercourse, boys or girls?

Having established the limits of a person's sexual activity, the epidemiologist then elicits the numbers of sexual contacts in a given period of time and determines their names. In the interview, the epidemiologist is interested in the critical period of 6 months prior to the appearance of symptoms.

Another series of questions used by the epidemiologist deals with the social-sexual community around the patient. The term "cluster interview" is used to describe this questioning concerning the sexual liaisons and interrelationships that exist between people in our society. In the cluster interview, the epidemiologist obtains from the patient a selected group of people who may be observed and studied for venereal infection.

The patient re-interview is an important phase in syphilis epidemiology. It helps develop incomplete information. Actually, a person who has named 5 contacts may give inadequate information about them. In the re-interview, he may give new information including the names of the 6th, 7th, or 8th contacts. The re-interview is done within 72 hours of the first. It serves to stimulate memory and to jog recall so that additional persons are named.

A contact is a person who has been sexually exposed to syphilis with information adequate for location.

The investigation involves the location of the contact and the choice of a physician or clinic. If the contact says, I wish to go to a private doctor, and is unable to afford the cost of care, there is an emergency medical fund which provides a set fee for the diagnosis and therapy of syphilis.

In talking with the contact and motivating him to seek a medical examination, the epidemiologist must discuss his or her sexual behavior and sexual activity. In this discussion, the epidemiologist attempts to determine other people with whom the contact may have been exposed. In this way, the chain of persons who may be brought to examination is enlarged.

In the cluster interview an infected man names a woman as a contact. She is found to be infected, too. She is interviewed and names the original patient, no one else. Obviously, there is something wrong; there has to be a third party in this chain of infection. The man is then asked how well he knows the woman, does he have other friends who know her, is there a possibility that his friends may have had sex with her, do any have lesions similar to his? In the cluster interview, the names of many persons may be obtained. All who are named are brought in for examination. The infected were treated and the noninfected were given epidemiological treatment.

The epidemiologist must assure that the contact or suspect is examined. Again, a complete oral, anal, genital, dermal examination is required and a speculum examination is very necessary.

Epidemiological treatment involves administration of a therapeutic dose of penicillin to sero-negative, asymptomatic, clinically negative contacts. In a well controlled study, conducted by the Public Health Service, 10 per cent of clinically negative, sero-negative contacts of primary-secondary syphilis developed lesions and transmitted the disease to 5 additional persons. In New Jersey we followed sero-negative, asymptomatic contacts of primary-secondary syphilis for 90 to 100 days and found that 30 per cent developed clinical lesions. We argue that many of the contacts are in the incubation stage of syphilis, and by applying a therapeutic dose of penicillin to sero-negative clinically negative contacts, we prevent the further development of syphilis and its transmission. At the present time, approximately 70 per cent of contacts are receiving epidemiological treatment from our private physicians and in our clinics. It has been said that if we can treat 30 per cent of all primary-secondary syphilis before the opportunity exists of transmission to another person in a matter of about 10 years we can eradicate syphilis.[6]

The results of the epidemiological investigations throughout the United States are combined by the Public Health Service. Contact interviews, re-interviews, and cluster interviews are evaluated and the yield of new cases is determined.

In the United States epidemiological activities were expanded to include interviewing of 91.8 per cent of reported infectious syphilis patients in fiscal year 1963 and 93.6 per cent of reported infectious patients in the first 9 months of fiscal year 1964. As a result of this activity 102,135 contacts of primary or secondary syphilis patients reported by clinics and 33,017 contacts of primary or secondary syphilis patients reported by private physicians were investigated in fiscal year 1963 and the first 9 months of fiscal year 1964. From these two groups 11,014 cases of primary-secondary syphilis were brought to treatment.[15]

During the first 10 months of fiscal year 1964, 47 states working with the federal government in venereal disease control projects were able to identify the probable source contact for 60.4 per cent of the primary and secondary syphilis patients interviewed. Spread cases among contacts were identified for 37.1 per cent of secondary patients interviewed as compared to 19.6 per cent of the primary patients interviewed.

Re-interviewing has been particularly responsible for improvement in the number of contacts elicited per patient. Nationally 1 out of every 5 contacts examined was obtained during a re-interview. Approximately 29 per cent of the re-interview contacts were infected and almost half of these contacts were brought to treatment.

A study of the concept of cluster interviewing in 1963 indicated the following. When a patient names a cluster suspect having symptoms similar to his own or those demonstrated through visual aids, the yield of new cases is often as great as from contacts of primary-secondary syphilis. When a patient is induced to discuss persons he thinks are sex partners or very close friends of other infectious people, 1 out of every 23 will require treatment.

When a patient is motivated to suggest that sex partners or close friends of his contact should be examined, 1 out of every 35 will require treatment.

This study and subsequent studies have demonstrated that contacts and suspects named by infectious persons have knowledge of other persons' behavior. This knowledge can quickly lead to other related group members who have syphilis.

Health department personnel throughout the United States

visited 62,406 physicians in 1963 and 88,326 in 1964 to enlist their cooperation in reporting cases of syphilis and permitting their patients to be interviewed. Private physician infectious syphilis reporting increased from 6827 cases in 1962 to 8498 cases in 1964. The major purposes of the physician program were to explain the need for better case reporting, to urge each physician to report his cases promptly and completely to the health department, and to enlist his cooperation in permitting his early syphilis patients to be interviewed for sex contacts by a trained interviewer from the health department. In addition, the visit includes a discussion of the increasing syphilis problem, the Public Health Control Program, and the diagnostic, epidemiological, and educational services available to the physician from the health department. Information indicating the effectiveness of visits to the private physician is available from Public Health Service statistics. For example, primary and secondary syphilis cases reported by private physicians are increasing in numbers at a much faster rate than cases reported by clinic physicians. The cases reported by private physicians account for an increasing proportion of the total early syphilis attack rate reported throughout the nation.

A steadily increasing percentage of infectious syphilis patients reported by private physicians is being interviewed for sex contacts by health department personnel. Such cases are thus included in the early syphilis epidemiology process which prevents further spread of infection.

A program of venereal disease information and education is taking shape, the like of which has never been seen before. Educational messages are finding their way to every corner of the land via press, radio, television, platform, and class room with one principal object, that the infected and potentially infected will recognize the personal threat and distinct possibility of being infected. That is, that their personal index of suspicion, their syphilis worry index, if you will, will become more sensitive. The effect, hopefully, will be to bring a significant number of exposed persons to examination at the earliest sign, or perhaps even in the absence of a sign.

In summary:

Primary-secondary syphilis constitutes an epidemic threat to the United States with over 22,000 cases reported in 1964.

There are an estimated one million cases of gonorrhea in the United States annually. The infectious venereal diseases are most prevalent in the age groups 15 to 19 and 20 to 24.

Primary-secondary syphilis has not been adequately reported by physicians, thus the search for sources of infection and persons to whom the disease may have spread has been prevented.

Every physician should be a part of the "primary-secondary sphilis epidemiological team," participating by diagnosing, reporting, and requiring the epidemiological investigation of his patients.

Epidemiological investigation requires patient interviewing and re-interviewing for sex contacts, contact location, examination, and interview.

All contacts should be treated because 10 per cent of sero-negative, clinically negative, sexual contacts of primary-secondary syphilis develop lesions and transmit disease.

Progress is being made:

Of reported infectious syphilis patients in the first 9 months of fiscal year 1964 93 per cent were interviewed for sex contacts.

The sources of syphilis and persons to whom it has been spread are being discovered with increasing and regular frequency among sex contacts of new cases.

A massive public and professional awareness program is being undertaken to raise the syphilis suspicion index.

REFERENCES

1. American Social Health Association: *Today's VD Control Problem*, p. 13. 1965.
2. American Social Health Association: *Today's VD Control Problem*, p. 14. 1965.
3. American Social Health Association: *Today's VD Control Problem*, p. 15. 1965.
4. American Social Health Association: *Today's VD Control Problem*, p. 19. 1965.
5. American Social Health Association: *Today's VD Control Problem*, p. 67. 1965.
6. Brown, W. J.: So far to go, so little time. U.S.P.H.S. Venereal Disease Seminar, Miami, 1964.
7. Brown, W. J.: Strategy of syphilis eradication. Speech, Southern Medical Association, Memphis, Tenn., 1964.

8. Committee on Public Health, The New York Academy of Medicine: Resurgence of venereal disease. Bull. New York Acad. Med., *40:* 802, 1964.
9. Curtis, A. C.: National survey of VD treatment. J. A. M. A., *186:* 46, 1963.
10. Moore, M. B.: Epidemiologic treatment of contacts of infectious syphilis. Pub. Health Rep., *78:* 966, 1963.
11. Parran, T.: *Shadow on the Land: Syphilis,* p. 247. Reynal and Hitchcock, New York, 1937.
12. U.S. Department of Health, Education, and Welfare: *Venereal Disease Branch Report,* p. 1. 1963–1964.
13. U.S. Department of Health, Education, and Welfare: *Venereal Disease Branch Report,* p. 2. 1963–1964.
14. U.S. Department of Health, Education, and Welfare: *Venereal Disease Branch Report,* p. 4. 1963–1964.
15. U.S. Department of Health, Education, and Welfare: *Venereal Disease Branch Report,* p. 7. 1963–1964.

10

The Psychological Impact of Pregnancy on the Adolescent Girl

Allen E. Marans, M.D.

I plan to approach the subject of "The Psychological Impact of Pregnancy on the Adolescent Girl" in two ways: first, to share with you in an impressionistic manner my experiences in working with pregnant girls who were 15 years or younger; and secondly to speculate on the bases for the difficulties encountered in the prenatal obstetrical management of this age group. My goal will be to present the details of the story which was so sensitively headlined by Marchetti and Menaker in 1950 as follows: "We're convinced from our observations that the most important consideration to be given the young pregnant girl lies in the management of her antepartum course. There are psychic as well as physical changes that must be borne in mind. The effect of the fear of pain, of reproach, of shame, of the anticipation of an ordeal and many other mental impacts to which she may be subjected, have to be managed with far more and somewhat different understanding." [13]

The city of Washington shares the situation being experienced universally [1, 2, 5, 7, 10-14] of an increasing frequency of pregnancy in young adolescents. The Maternal and Child Health Division of the District of Columbia Health Department has long been concerned with the problem of providing appropriate and adequate prenatal care for this difficult age group. As part of this effort an interview with a social worker was an automatic requirement for every girl 15 years or under on her first visit to the Health Department maternity clinics. (The age was lowered from 16 in 1960 when the social workers found that more cases than they could handle were being referred.) I was afforded the opportunity from September, 1962, through September, 1963, to serve as psychiatric consultant to the social workers aiding these girls and to work with a number of them directly.

There were roughly 10 to 15 new patients referred on the basis of their age each week. More than three-fourths of these had multiple visits with the social workers or me during the remainder of their pregnancies. The vast majority of these girls were 15 years of age although there was a fair number of 14 year olds. The youngest was 12, but these and the 13 year olds comprised but a small fraction of the sample I will describe. The population served by the clinic is of the lower socio-economic group and predominantly Negro.

The most frequent source of referral to the clinic was the Public Health school nurse. (The majority were still in junior high school.) The pregnancy would be brought to the nurse's attention most often by the physical education teachers. Sharp-eyed and alerted to the significance of rapid body changes, the gym teachers pride themselves on detecting early pregnancies among their students. Of course in many cases the mother brought her daughter for care before the condition came to the school's attention.

These young girls made attempts to conceal their pregnancy as long as possible from parents, authorities, friends, and also from themselves. The undesirable reality was resisted well into the last trimester in several cases. One girl steadfastly maintained through her eighth month of pregnancy that she had never had intercourse. A 13-year-old girl argued rather pathetically that she hadn't engaged in sexual intercourse since she was 7 years old. I think we could safely say that the unconscious process of denial had the fullest cooperation of the conscious wish, that things were not the way they so very much seemed to be.

The diagnosis of pregnancy made unofficially but usually with certainty by the mother at home caused some immediate results.

The dread with which the girl anticipated this confrontation was not lessened by familiarity within the same situation as experienced by classmates, her neighborhood acquaintances, or even her older siblings, or even by the fact that she herself may have been conceived by her mother under very similar circumstances. She faced her mother's and father's anger with shame and guilt. There is no question about the intensity of each girl's remorse despite the apparently successful efforts of some to appear unconcerned. One girl stopped writing to her father rather than confess her condition. The fact that he was in prison did not diminish her reaction.

Despite her more violent initial response, the mother was likely to become tolerant sooner than the father. The frequently heard statement by the female relatives after angrily expressing their disappointment was, "Everybody is entitled to one mistake, but don't let it happen again." They would ask in frustration, "Do you want to end up like me with 10 kids?" Yet it was not uncommon for a mother to arrange the traditional baby shower for her daughter toward the end of the pregnancy with warmth and expectant happiness. The father more often evidenced a permanent change in his relationship with his daughter.

Occasionally the boyfriend will bravely confess his role to his and the girl's parents. He may offer marriage (even though he may only be a few years older and still far from finishing high school), or he may offer promises of financial support or his parents' willingness to share or entirely care for the baby. These offers are usually met with rejection by the girl's mother and the admonition that he better never see her daughter again. Sometimes the relationship is allowed to continue with the "understanding" that there will be no more intercourse. One such case demonstrates the typical pattern of the latter variety. A 15-year-old primigravida was attentively squired each and every visit to the maternity clinic through the second and well into the third trimester by her 16-year-old boyfriend. He promised that right after the football season he would get an after-school job and begin buying things for the baby to be. Well, he made the track team. The implementation of his good intention was further delayed. As our patient in her last trimester got more and more uncomfortable and less and less romantically or even socially inclined, she saw less and less of her formerly devoted boyfriend. After the baby was born, though the patient had moved in with *his* sisters to watch all their children so they could work, his visits to the baby, much less to her, became far less frequent. Then she discovered he had begun dating another girl.

Getting back to the immediate results of the girl's state of pregnancy being known, there are of course social as well as parental reactions. As soon as the school authorities become officially aware of the diagnosis, the student must cease school attendance. It is a rule in the District of Columbia that the principal of the school is the one who will decide whether the girl shall be permitted to return to that school after the baby is born or whether she will be transferred to another. Almost invariably if the girl does return to school, she is transferred to a new setting. This is usually the girl's wish too. The school authorities do not wish to take a position which might seem to condone pregnancy in the "student body." Many principals fear that the pregnant girl or young mother in the school might become a model for emulation by her impressionable classmates. The school authorities are quite concerned with the plight of these unfortunate girls and constant efforts are being made to improve the handling of this difficult problem.

The District of Columbia school system does provide visiting teachers on a once or twice a week basis for pregnant students. Additionally, through the combined efforts of the Board of Education, the Welfare Department, and the Health Department, a school for pregnant girls has been established where continuing education, health supervision, and preparation for motherhood is available to a limited number. However, the waiting list is long though the school is less than 2 years old. This is a needed step in the right direction though. It has become evident that because it is already an overextended program which cannot provide adequate time for each student, the home bound teaching has met with less than desired results. Often poor students to begin with, the infrequency of contact with a teacher plus the lethargy and impatience associated with pregnancy and the almost exclusive preoccupation with herself and her pregnancy preclude much of an investment in academic pursuit. It is much easier to daydream about becoming a nurse or cosmetologist than to contemplate the actual steps of keeping up with school work and being better prepared to return.

The social isolation felt by some of the young primigravidae is one of the most disturbing features of their condition to them. We have seen that they are excluded (except for the fortunate few who get into the special school) from the main focus of teen-age activity, the school. A few of their intimate girlfriends may drop by to see them or call them on the phone in the beginning but this occurs with rapidly decreasing frequency the longer they are removed from what is going on in their peer world. Parents usually warn their children to stay away from such a girl as though her dreaded state were directly contagious. This gets transmitted to the patient and enhances her feelings of guilt and loneliness. Often though, the pregnancy becomes a status symbol and gains for the girl an envious and loyal following of interested girlfriends; or, the pregnancy gives her entrée to the group of young mothers who are seen as being more sophisticated than their uninitiated peers. Even so, there is a relative isolation when a girl is not participating in the school-centered teen-age world.

As demonstrated earlier, even the rare boyfriend who is staunchly loyal has his breaking off point. In the majority of cases the disappointment with a boyfriend comes much earlier. Usually as soon as he finds out she is pregnant, he stops seeing her. Almost invariably though, he wants to see his baby soon after it is born. On the girl's part, there is often disgust with, and hatred of, the amorous suitor toward whom there had probably been marked ambivalence before the deed was done. Undoubtedly there is the projection of her sense of guilt but also there is the expectation of abandonment which turns her away from her former partner. Whether the boyfriend rejects her, or *vice versa*, the evidence of the girl's sexual availability often attracts boys who hope to pick her up on the rebound. "I'll accept you with your baby" is often the promise used to obtain safe sex. These lonely girls are easy prey and thus expose themselves to further disappointment and further loss of self-esteem.

The isolation aspects of her confinement are further enhanced by her partially imagined but also realistic expectations that "the word" will spread even more quickly than the contours of her figure. By the third trimester, everyone will look at her and say or think, "We know what you've been doing." The adults as well as the children in the neighborhood to her mind seem to delight in the young girl's mortification, so she avoids them by staying in the house.

Among the more extroverted girls, there were some who continued going to movies and parties through most of their pregnancy. Dancing, though, could prove to be physically as well as emotionally embarrassing to the enlarged girl in view of the dexterity and energy required for the current adolescent addictions. The refreshments served at parties were all likely to be on the obstetrician's unapproved list as probable contributors to the increased incidence of toxemia found in young adolescents. Marchetti and Menaker[13] described the "jitterbug diet" which consisted of Coca-Cola or Pepsi-Cola, salted peanuts, potato chips, and hot dogs. To make this current, we need merely to change the name to "the young twisters' diet" and add pizza. As one girl put it, "What's the fun of going to a party if you can't do the wild dances or enjoy the food!"

Thus we see that there are combinations of social, physical, and emotional deprivations in operation which contribute to the isolation of the young adolescent during her pregnancy. Whole sets of age adequate behavior patterns formulated and tested by the group are unavailable to nonparticipants, yet peer relationships are essential to the development of appropriate identifications that are so necessary in the consolidation of self-concepts and achievement of a healthy measure of independence.[9] Whether, as young unmarried mothers, these girls are ever able to regain a place in the mainstream of appropriate adolescent interaction and development is open to question.

As if these weren't enough burdens for a 12- to 15-year-old girl there are also the usual fears of childbirth which become compounded by youth. There were concerns familiar to the obstetricians working with adult primigravidae. Many were afraid they wouldn't be able to stand the pains of the delivery. Most were afraid they wouldn't know when they were in labor. Many were afraid they wouldn't get to the hospital in time and they would have the baby on the street or in a taxicab. Some were afraid they would go to the hospital and be sent home because they weren't ready. Many were afraid they would get to the hospital, and it would be the right time, and they would have to stay. Most were afraid of the doctors and what they would do to them. Almost uniformly they dreaded the possibility of spinal anesthesia because "it leaves you paralyzed." They were concerned with the after-effects of the pregnancy on their bodies. "Will my stomach ever get back to its right size?" "Will the big veins in my legs always be that way now?" "I don't want to breast feed because that leaves your breasts ugly."

Additionally there were fears which seemed peculiar to this age group. Some were afraid they weren't big enough, that is, either they would burst as the baby grew, or the baby would grow so big it wouldn't be able to get out, and it then might grow to their insides and they would die. Others stated rather poignantly that they might die during childbirth just because they were too young to be having babies, their bodies weren't ready for it.

Although these fears originated in the mind of each girl they were frequently augmented by stories from well meaning female friends, neighbors, and relatives. These usually gruesome stories were of a rather primitive variety and were used to demonstrate the dire outcome if some favorite prohibition were not heeded. It was not surprising that these externally inspired fears were dissipated by a brief discussion with the social workers or me much more readily than those which originated within the individual unless, of course, as frequently happened, they did coincide.

Some of the fears were iatrogenically reinforced intentionally in hopes of achieving more cooperation from the patient. The outstanding example of this had to do with the problem of weight gain. In an attempt to induce the adolescents to curb their appetites and avoid "the young twisters diet," grave prognostications were spelled out in frightening detail. This usually resulted in at best a temporary cessation of the continuous progress of exaggerated weight gain. Often an effect of the opposite intended was brought about.

The pathogenesis of adolescent prenatal overeating was seen as follows: (1) the impetus to appetite common to pregnancy met with no resistance in these girls long accustomed to irregular family eating patterns; (2) confinement to the home alone permitted a constant proximity to an unguarded food supply; (3) lack of adequate gratification from the other teen-age activities added to a low threshold for frustration tolerance and served to intensify her need for impulse relief in the available form of eating; and (4) eating became a way of relieving all emotional discomforts—unhappiness, guilt, anxiety, and fear. Augmented by the inactivity of the last few months, weight gain and worrying were closely related. A difficult but gratifying experience was the reduction of eating for the remainder of the pregnancy which followed the relief of fears and anxieties through enlightening discussions in several cases.

Another source of difficulty for the majority of the young mothers-to-be during their pregnancies resulted from the looseness of their family structures. The stable family with parents married and both living in the home was present in less than a third of the cases. The remainder presented a variety of situations few of which provided for the heightened needs of the frightened, guilty, isolated young adult. It was the rare home which presented a framework of rules which could have led to the self-discipline which might have prevented the pregnancy or facilitated acquiescence to the necessary dietary restrictions.

Many of these youngsters had been reared by a succession of relatives in frequently shifting settings. There were few of these relatives who were willing to continue such care after the pregnancy was discovered and the shame had to be faced. Then it was time to send the girl back to her mother who may have been unable to keep her in the first place because, for example: (1) she had married a man other than the girl's father and he didn't want the young girl around; or (2) there was inadequate money or room for all of her children so the mother had kept the youngest with her and had gotten relatives to take in the older children who could help out around the house; or (3) the mother may have been so young when this child was born that the grandmother raised her—that is until this girl turned out to be "bad" like her mother.

There were innumerable other such circumstances all of which were conducive to the development of feelings of rejection and worthlessness, and anger toward the one who had deserted them —mother. The tearful, angry confrontations between some daughters and mothers which occurred during joint interviews clearly demonstrated the dearth of solace that would be derived from those relationships at that point. The mother once recovered from her anger at the girl as mentioned earlier could forgive, probably on the basis of identification with her daughter in such a familiar difficulty. In some cases, however, too much disappointment had occurred in their young lives for these girls even in their time of great need to trust their mothers enough to depend on them for help. Though yearning for a closeness, they often forego the opportunity the mother presents. There is suggestive evidence that they thus deprive themselves in an attempt to maintain their sense of independence which may have been such an important defense against the lack of security that they have had to endure.

Thus far, I have presented material derived in the privacy of the social casework or psychiatric interview situation after some trust has been established. These girls often present themselves quite differently to the rest of the maternity clinic staff. They may act indifferent, unconcerned, and even proud. Or they may assume immature and irresponsible attitudes and seem surprised that anything is expected of them, even information or cooperation. In view of the role the clinic plays in removing the last vestige of hope that she is not pregnant, it is not hard to understand why the young teen-ager might face her prenatal visits with other than optimal attitudes. Of course there are other contributing factors some of which arise in response to the very nature of the clinic experience.

To be examined in the clinic, the minor needs her parent's written consent. This means of course that the confrontation with the mother as discussed previously will have already occurred. The mother must then bring her daughter to the clinic and face her shame openly. In addition to this discomfort, there is the inconvenience of the clinic hours and long wait which may rekindle the anger felt toward her daughter. This is very often dealt with by the mother's making clinic attendance a punitive measure, as if to say "see what you've gotten yourself into."

The mother frequently assumes a hypermoralistic approach with the staff in the daughter's presence in an attempt to dissociate herself from her daughter's guilt. In so doing she presents her daughter in the worse possible light and often induces some of the maternity clinic staff to rebuke the friendless, defenseless girl for letting her mother down. This, of course, deprives the mother of the tolerance and acceptance that she is seeking for herself since she cannot really overcome the sense of responsibility for her child's actions. The staff member thus loses the opportunity to help mother and daughter face the unpleasant reality in a more mutually supportive manner.

The first order of business on an introductory visit to the maternity clinic was the completion of the important forms by the Public Assistance Division worker to determine eligibility for clinic services. The adolescents usually reacted to requests for information about the "putative father," his willingness to pay, etc. defensively. Under the guise of "I don't know" answers, she could avoid giving incriminating evidence to a representative of the law. At the same time she might be retaliating for the discomfort she was being caused by such questions, by withholding the information that the worker needed. That she was capable of inducing a negative response to herself by the clinic staff often became apparent to the pregnant adolescent girl in her first contact. This could be used as collaborative evidence for her anticipation that the clinic would be a hostile and dangerous place.

Medical record data had to be obtained next. Specific information about herself and the "putative father" had to be yielded to another unknown person regarding the very personal situation of being pregnant without a husband and at such a young age. It would be mentioned at this point by the clerk that copies of these records would go to the hospital where she would have her baby delivered. The protection of privacy was no longer available.

The need for privacy was also expressed in the extreme modesty which became manifested when urine samples were requested and after the change from street clothes to examining gowns was made. Attitudes evidenced during height and weight checks and while waiting to be called for examination by the doctors were more to be expected in chaste convent school girls than sexually experienced young women. This might be attributed solely to the shame of the condition which they were still trying to hide. However, on closer examination it was noted to be merely an exaggeration of the modesty concerns of the older members of the clinic population of the same socio-economic-educational background.

Prudery, obviously inconsistent in view of their pregnant state, seemed to be the rule rather than the exception among this group.

For the 12 through 15 year olds there was another contributor to this extreme modesty. The giving over of body products and the abandonment of the protection of street clothes seemed to place these young girls in a frighteningly exposed and submissive position. The examination by the physician in their minds had become a dreaded assault on their body.

Anxiety in the presence of a strange physician is certainly not unexpected, but add to this the feeling created by the moment of truth when all wishful doubts about her true state of being pregnant are removed. Add to that the position of authority of the physician and the attitudes of angry censure for her condition which she expects from authority figures. Add to that her embarrassing experiences in the clinic thus far which may not have inspired any confidence that she will be dealt with in a sensitive manner. Also add to that the friendless, isolated, defenseless, helpless feelings encountered so frequently among these girls. Add to that the fear of the physician as one who creates pain by needles and examinations especially when he examines one's most sensitive areas, the anatomy of which may be so vaguely understood. That this examination could be, and commonly is, seen as a sexual assault should not be surprising. It then becomes understandable that the anxiety may be so great that it may generalize and produce exaggerated responses to even blood pressure measurements, very likely to the obtaining of blood samples, and quite likely to even the gentlest handling of the pelvic examination. The same response to anxiety and wish to retaliate as occurred with the Public Assistance Division worker may appear here, that is, an inability to supply necessary information, for example, date of last menstrual period, date of menarche, etc. and an inability to comply with the simplest request for cooperation, for example, keeping her feet in the stirrups, etc.

The clinic obstetrician so accustomed to dealing with adults, many of whom are multiparous, most of whom have had previous pelvic examinations, usually finds these frightened, uncooperative youngsters both pathetic and frustrating. Pressed by the large number of other patients to be seen, he was only occasionally able to spend as much time with each 12 through 15 year old as he thought she really needed. There was another pressure to which the obstetricians responded. Moral issues aside, these girls were seen to be in serious trouble. There were already the handicaps of their lower socio-economic class origins. Problems of survival, much less enhancing their chances for betterment, pre-existed the pregnancy. The precocious pregnancy was seen as a final overwhelming reality regarding which the obstetricians had grave doubts that they could be of any help. They were only too glad to turn over these "impossible" cases to the social worker or me as quickly as possible. There seemed to be a wish that our vaguely understood techniques possessed a magical quality which would allow us to effect great changes in these girls.

Despite their doubts and without their being fully aware of the difficult task they had accomplished, the obstetricians helped the girls through their physical examinations in the majority of instances with only minor manifestations of anxiety breaking through. I will return to the importance of the function of the physician later.

The obstetricians usually gave the necessary instructions regarding prenatal care and further schedules of appointments in a succinct fashion directly to the girl and then referred her on to the Public Health Nurse member of the clinic team for more complete particulars. The relief which she felt when she left the doctor's office was short lived as her mother rejoined her in the conference with the nurse. A common situation was one in which every instruction given to the patient by the nurse would be punctuated by the mother's comments. "You hear that." "Ha, you won't be able to do that anymore." "You better pay attention to what the nurse is telling you if you know what is good for you." The daughter's face would grow longer and longer and the set of her jaw would become more resolute. There would be no response to the nurse's statements and almost never any questions when they were solicited.

As mentioned previously, the nurse might join the mother against the uncooperative patient, but another reaction was also demonstrated. Identification with the patient in her struggle with the critical mother was fostered by the commonly held attitude that this child was in her present mess because of inadequate interest and inadequate supervision on the part of the mother.

Thus nurses not infrequently found themselves impelled to come to the defense of the girls even to the point of manifesting critical attitudes towards the mother. However, the view of the nurse as a judgmental and potentially critical person was formed by the girl regardless of whose side the nurse took when she did take a side. It was when the nurse was able to demonstrate respect for both parties and facilitate a mutual understanding for mother and daughter that she became most useful and most used.

The importance of the girl's attitude toward the nurse member of the maternity clinic team became apparent. There were also visiting health nurses, school nurses, nurses in the hospital where she would go to have the baby, and nurses in the well-baby clinics where she would bring her baby. The expectations derived from her experience with the maternity clinic nurses were readily transferred to the other nursing groups and became either a source of comfort and reassurance or a reinforcement of the lonely and frightened feeling she harbored.

The nurses, in appreciation of the importance of their role, felt pressured to give these young girls as much as possible to prepare them for their ordeal of pregnancy and delivery and to prevent a recurrence of the condition. In response to the patient's passivity and under doctors' orders, very often the nurse pumped in far more education than she knew the girl could handle at that point. An example of this was the practice of making referrals to postpartum Planned Parenthood Clinics at the time of the first prenatal visit. To insure that the importance of this far off step was appreciated, the nurse would launch into a lecture on the mechanics of diaphragm utilization, replete with multicolored drawings and sample devices. After the nurses and doctors had an opportunity to reflect on this routine, they quickly abandoned the diaphragm demonstration and with much relief used the time to address more currently pertinent issues.

With the feeling of "having had it and then some," the youngest group in the maternity clinic then had interviews with the social workers or in a limited number of instances with me. Some responded to the friendly interest shown in them with characteristic passivity. Many, though, experienced an overflowing of their pent up fears, conflicts, and anger regarding themselves, their pregnancy, their relationships with family members, their relationship with boyfriends, etc., etc., etc. These and subsequent such interviews allowed in many cases the opportunity to discuss fears and plans for both present and the future. Some girls could never be "reached" in this way. Among these, successes were often scored by the visiting nurse or visiting teacher, perhaps thus indicating that some girls needed more "reaching out to."

One of the questions the social workers and I routinely posed to a number of the 12- to 15-year-old primigravidae was, "What do you think would be the biggest problem to a young girl who is pregnant?" The answers fell into two categories. One had to do with the fear of isolation or abandonment by parents, boyfriends, or friends. The other concerned their physical condition and the threat to it which their pregnancy posed. I would now like to amplify my experience and thoughts regarding the latter not only because of its impact on the pregnant girl but also because of its implications on the more usual course of adolescence.

As details were being obtained about the fears these girls had regarding being pregnant at their age, another type of reaction evidenced itself. Repeatedly, there were comments to the effect that they didn't feel or act "like themselves." They couldn't "control their tempers" like they used to be able to do. They had become "selfish." They were "changed," "different." As they thought about why they felt and acted differently, two answers stood out. One was the fear of having the baby. The other was the change in their bodies.

The latter was well described by one girl in this way, "When your body feels different, you feel different." Others talked about the strange sensation of not really knowing their body boundaries, "Like moving into a new house and not knowing where things are." For example, they grossly misjudged necessary clothing size. They bumped into things with their enlarged abdomens and breasts. They were constantly being amazed at their appearance in the mirror. The possibility that this sort of reaction could be wishful thinking that they were not different, that is, not pregnant, cannot be completely ruled out, but other evidence makes this unlikely. When they were asked if they had ever experienced anything like this before they all answered in the affirmative without hesitation. Of course, this was the way they had felt when they had begun to develop sexually.

Thus, the strangeness they felt had as a very major component the rapid physical changes they were experiencing as the result of their being pregnant. Caplan[6] has talked about puberty, pregnancy, and menopause as normally occurring critical periods of development. During each of these periods a state of disequilibrium (like Erikson's "identity diffusion"[8]) occurs which then allows for a reconstitution at a more mature level of functioning. It was impressive that more serious consequences did not result from the superimposing of one such identity crisis so closely upon another.

Bibring and associates,[3,4] in their study of the psychological processes in pregnancy among a group of fairly normal adult primigravidae, found a narcissistic period occurring in the early stages of pregnancy which manifested itself among other things as an intensification of interest in the woman's own body. In these older women, the focus later shifted from the process of the pregnancy to the product, that is, the baby. Interest in the forthcoming baby's physical condition then governed her thinking and this represented an important step in personality maturation, that is the woman was becoming a mother. This step did not occur to the same degree in the adolescent mother-to-be. She remained primarily narcissistic. Her baby was seen as a possession, a doll, rather than a human being distinct from herself.

Thus, we see 12- to 15-year-old girls who have yet to complete the reconstitution from the critical period of puberty and who find themselves undergoing another state of disorganization. To make it worse, there are few of the patterns of society supporting her through the new threat to her physical-psychical well-being. We have heard of two of her reactions in our population—withdrawal into lonely isolation, and passive resistance which so often incurs the wrath rather than the support of others. I have alluded to a third and far more magical, maladaptive, yet understandable means of coping—the wishful thinking, the denial of unpleasant reality that is neurotic rather than of psychotic proportions.

It is the denial of reality which enables these young girls, often abetted by parents and boyfriends, to make grandiose plans for the baby and a happy life thereafter with utter disregard for the facts and their real probabilities. The decreased frustration tolerance, which may have contributed to their becoming pregnant in the first place, also makes facing their situation realistically in order to formulate constructive approaches less possible. The denial is a way out.

To help these girls forego the denial, it seemed necessary to relieve the sources of anxiety which perpetuated it, and to demonstrate that facing the reality could be more permanently helpful, if not gratifying. The girls were encouraged to verbalize their fears in detail to the point at which misconceptions in anatomy, physiology, and the process of pregnancy became apparent even to them. They were asked to draw pictures of their insides and the baby and the process of delivery for example. As their confusion became evident, they were able to ask for information which they seemed to assimilate. I might add here that when they were asked what they thought was the cause of the pain during labor, the majority said it was the baby kicking and moving trying to get out. These thoughts are certainly not conducive to positive feelings about one's offspring.

I cannot prove that such efforts at helping these girls become more familiar with their bodies and the processes taking place in them aided in the consolidation of their identities. A more efficient and more effective means of practicing such an approach would be achieved by the formation of small groups for such discussions on a regular basis. (Since my time in the clinic this practice has been developed and has resulted in a better than 90 per cent clinic attendance rate for this age group.) I do feel that even in the individual sessions the girls were impressed with the fact that there were people in the community who could be turned to when problems presented.

Another way of helping these girls face reality so that they could be better prepared to deal with it was to arrange for prenatal group visits to the municipal hospital where they would be delivered. This had a double effect. The girls who were willing to go (and not all were) became familiar with the physical setup, the people, and the routines they would encounter. The hospital staff was made more aware of the special problems these girls presented and their needs for special handling. The hospital staff members say they can differentiate without prior knowledge, but solely on the basis of their behavior during labor, which of this age group had the prenatal visit and which did not. The prenatal hospital visit is frequently used by middle class, more mature expectant mothers who have above average capacity for abstract reasoning. Such an actual experience would seem to be far more essential to a group more dependent for solving problems of concreteness in their thought processes.

An additional dividend of the hospital visit was derived from the clinic nurse being the group leader for the trip and introducing the girls individually to the hospital nurse. The ubiquity of nurses previously mentioned facilitates the development of the concept that the nurse is a community resource readily available and dependable in time of need.

From the foregoing, I am sure that it is also apparent that in my estimation the obstetrician is in an ideal position to provide information that will lessen the impact of the bodily changes on the young girl's already precarious self-image. By explicitly predicting step by step each bodily reaction to the pregnancy, the obstetrician provides a well marked map. As each landmark appears and is recognized as promised, the young pregnant traveler develops more confidence in the map and the map maker, and the conviction grows that the journey will end safely because she has been helped to know who and where she is.

In conclusion, I have no illusions that I have covered in a complete fashion the "Psychological Impact of Pregnancy on the Adolescent Girl." Nor do I wish to imply that some of the simple measures we attempted are anything but a beginning to the provision of really appropriate and adequate services for these girls. I do hope that I have contributed to the store of "more and somewhat different understanding" that Dr. Marchetti called for in 1950.[13]

I would like to express my gratitude to Mrs. Harryette Dixon, Miss Rachael Geiger, and Mrs. Marion Groce, the social workers who shared their girls, their thoughts, and their work with me. I am likewise indebted to Dr. Samuel Shwartz, Chief of the Bureau of Maternal and Child Health of the District of Columbia

Department of Public Health, and to the entire staff of the maternity clinic whose cooperation made this study possible.

REFERENCES

1. Anzar, R., and Bennett, A. E.: Pregnancy in the adolescent girl. Am. J. Obst. & Gynec., *81:* 934, 1961.
2. Battaglia, F. C., Todd, M. F., and Hellgers, A. E.: Obstetric and pediatric complications of juvenile pregnancy. Pediatrics, *32:* 902, 1963.
3. Bibring, G.: Some considerations of the psychological processes in pregnancy. In *Psychoanalytic Study of the Child*, Vol. XIV. International Universities Press, Inc., New York, 1959.
4. Bibring, G., Dwyer, T. F., Huntington, D. S., Valenstein, A. F.: A study of the psychological processes in pregnancy and of the earliest mother-child relationship. In *Psychoanalytic Study of the Child*, Vol. XVI, p. 9. International Universities Press, Inc., New York, 1961.
5. Bochner, K.: Pregnancies in juveniles. Am. J. Obst. & Gynec., *83:* 269, 1962.
6. Caplan, G.: Recent trends in preventive child psychiatry. In *Emotional Problems of Early Childhood*, edited by G. Caplan. Basic Books, Inc., New York, 1955.
7. Clamon, A. D., and Bell, H. M.: Pregnancy in the very young teenager. Am. J Obst. & Gynec., *9:* 350, 1964.
8. Erikson, E. H.: Identity and the life cycle. Psychological Issues, Vol. 1, No. 1. International Universities Press, Inc., New York, 1959.
9. Hollingshead, A. B.: A sociologic perspective on adolescence. Pediat. Clin. North America, *7:* 131, 1960.
10. Hulka, J. F., and Schaaf, B. A.: Obstetrics in adolescents: a controlled study of deliveries by mothers 15 years of age and under. Obst. & Gynec., *23:* 678, 1964.
11. Israel, S. L., and Wontersz, T. B.: Teen-age obstetrics. Am. J. Obst. & Gynec., *85:* 659, 1963.
12. Israel, S. L., and Deutschberger, J.: Relation of the mother's age to obstetric performance. Obst. & Gynec., *24:* 411, 1964.
13. Marchetti, A. A., and Menaker, J. S.: Pregnancy and the adolescent. Am. J. Obst. & Gynec., *59:* 1013, 1950.
14. Mussio, T. J.: Primigravidas under age 14. Am. J. Obst. & Gynec., *84:* 442, 1962.

11

Sex Education in Adolescence

Sidney L. Werkman, M.D.

In years past sexuality in teen-agers was a dangerous issue to consider. That period seems to be part of history now. We don't have to justify the importance of sex education to ourselves, though we do to the general public. We are in a time of open discussion of sexuality, a time in which most of the issues are before the public, whether we are interested in having them there or not. In many ways physicians are behind the public in being concerned about sexuality. We have a mandate through medicine, and from education and the general society, for dealing with the great changes and ferment in sexuality, and we must find a way to make a most effective use of that mandate.

Parents are usually assigned the major responsibility for educating their children about sexuality. As we know from medical and psychiatric experience, they often misinform or underinform their children and greatly welcome help from the outside. As a matter of fact, parents quite regularly expect the physician to take over the job of describing to their children the physiology as well as the psychology of sexuality. As we will see later, this expectation is often not realized in a practical way. The issue, as in other private concerns, might end here if it were not that a great many of the results of sexuality impinge upon the general community. We have a major responsibility in preventive medicine and preventive mental hygiene before us.

In 1963 in Washington, D. C., there were 1600 illegitimate births in girls from 15 to 19 and 118 illegitimate babies in girls less than 15. About 40 per cent of young women who get married in the United States are pregnant at the time of their marriage. Venereal disease has just been discussed *in extenso* and is naturally an important concern in the mounting sex education program. But perhaps of greatest importance to us in the general field of medicine is that of mental hygiene—the anxiety and difficulties that teen-agers go through in thinking and dealing with sexuality, and the great burden of anxiety and unhappiness in later life that stems from early uncertainty or distortions about sexuality.

For example, a group of high school students were asked to state the questions they had about sex.[2] Here are their responses!

"What is petting? Is there anything wrong with petting? What do you do if the girl seems willing to go through with it? How can you tell a boy he's gone far enough? What part do boys play in girls' having babies? What is meant by contraceptives? Could you explain about abortion? Can venereal disease be spread by necking? Explain homosexuality, its causes and results. How can a girl tell if she's fit for married life? Is it true that girls mature faster than boys?"

Each of these questions could begin an extended discussion about facts, data, anxiety and uncertainty, family relationships, and the entire direction of life. In my own psychiatric work with patients, I have heard of many expressions of misinformation which create disturbances in teen-agers. Some of these disturbances have eaten away and festered for many months and years. For example, one girl told me that when she was 14, (I saw the girl at the age of 19) another girl had told her that she had to have intercourse with her father before she could make love with anyone else. This is a comment of a totally irresponsible, inflammatory kind. My patient had harbored the thought for 5 years, never certain whether to believe it or not. This is an aspect of many of the so-called facts, many of the concerns that teen-agers have. They think that they are not so, and yet they are not sure of it. And when the inflammatory material is not countered by direct statement, by an openness of discussion, the misinformation tends to take over. As we know, propaganda and rumor spread much faster than fact. This girl refused to kiss boys whom she liked or to be involved with them at all despite being attractive and previously quite socially interested. Her life was made miserable by this one bit of misinformation.

Another girl, not a psychiatric problem *per se*, had become involved in intercourse without knowing exactly what had occurred. She had had very little preparation for this and was the partner of a much more experienced and sophisticated boy. When she discovered what had actually happened, she became most distraught and further developed the idea, which she had heard in a casual way previously, that, in her words, "Once you had had sex, you wanted more and more." She was frightened that her downfall had occurred and that everyone would know that she was no longer a virgin.

If to these two vignettes are added the concerns of frigid, rejecting wives, and impotent or thoughtless husbands, people who have become involved in sexuality and marriage without a reasonable knowledge of the physiological and sexual aspects of their relationship, the task we have before us today is an impressive one.

The question is not, to paraphrase James Thurber, "Is sex (education) necessary?" but rather how it can be most effectively and helpfully offered to teen-agers. The question actually reaches into the years before adolescence, though I won't attempt to discuss this issue at length. The younger child, as you know, is exceedingly curious about pregnancy, birth, and anatomical aspects of the body, and there should be provision in one or another of the educational efforts made with children to supply them with accurate information about these questions. Otherwise they develop their own theories, their own distortions, which are always wild and disturbed in comparison to what the reasonable data are.

One of the questions that always comes up about sexual education is "Can it be harmful?" Of course it can. The willful distortion of sexual information given by adults, be they physicians or health educators, can continue to disturb a child's view of himself for a great period of time. Overtly or even covertly, seductive activities or encouragements toward perverse or anxiety-producing sexual activity are dangerous. More frequent a danger, however, is the giving of too little information together with veiled injunctions and frightened statements. For example, the physician who tells the youngster that masturbation is not bad, but that healthy, strong boys would not masturbate or would conquer the habit, confuses rather than educates. The greatest concern adults have about giving information to teen-agers is that it will be exciting to them and encourage them into further sexuality. However, when information is given reasonably and directly, there is no evidence that such stimulation occurs. This same argument has been advanced in regard to political and economic theories and has been discarded, and should be, along with other such ostrich-like views. Of paramount importance in giving sexual education is the fact that we are in a sexual revolution at the present time. Sexuality is becoming more free and increasingly distorted and unregulated among adolescents. The whole gamut of entertainment and communications media bombard the public with sexually exciting material that contains in it very little comment on values and norms. And it seems to me that if ever there was a time for stock taking and definitive statements by physicians, this is the time. Involvement with the sexual concerns and needs of teenagers can help the physician to do that very stock taking and make the venture an exceedingly contributing one for him as well as a useful one for teenagers.

One would think that the next step would be setting up a means for educating teenagers with the knowledge we have as physicians. But are doctors expert on sex? A study of medical students by Dr. Howard Lief of Tulane[3] suggests that we are not. He found that medical students knew a great deal about the anatomy and physiology of the sexual apparatus but little about the psychological or attitudinal aspects of sex. It was his opinion that the medical student comes to medical school with the same misconceptions, misinformation, and anxiety that people of a similar socio-economic background have. Only a few medical schools in this country teach students regularly about sexuality. Urology, obstetrics, and physiology cover certain aspects of sexuality, but there is little teaching about the intimate physiology of sexual excitement, the sexual background of intercourse, sexual adjustment and maladjustment, and marital adjustment and disharmony. Lief reports that, "without exception the doctors said the amount of instruction was most inadequate." The physicians said they had received no instruction at all concerning marital maladjustment and marital disharmony. One of the physicians responding said, "Information obtained in medical school came only from incidental considerations. It seems the professional staff was as negligent as the parents they so often condemn." Physicians responding stated that normal aspects of sex were almost completely avoided but the abnormal aspects received better coverage by the teaching staff. Sandler,[4] in another study, stated of medical students in Great Britain, "Probably less than half of the students of these schools have had anything like adequate sex instruction before they enter their professional lives."

It seems that we start from a shaky basis if we assume that physicians are effectively prepared to teach about sexuality. However, let us assume that we are talking about other people and we know all about it here. How and where can you teach most effectively and economically? You can work in a number of ways—through parent education, through education courses in the school, and through individual contacts with teen-agers. I think most of us would prefer to work through parents, for, historically, they have the primary role in this process. One method that has been used very successfully is to gather groups of parents together on a number of occasions and discuss the various aspects of sexuality. This mode of approach should be considered carefully as even the most sophisticated approaches to children from other sources are often doomed because of parents' conflicting ideas and emotionally tinged feelings that counteract the often healthy information given to the youngsters. Unfortunately, parents don't want to talk to their children about sex and they turn to outside help. And they seem to be unwilling to take the responsibility on their shoulders again. However, it is possible for physicians to begin to place that responsibility back on their shoulders, to educate them to the value and strength and satisfaction of assuming that responsibility.

Perhaps the most readily used mode of communication about sexuality is through school health courses. A profession of health educators has grown up in many school systems throughout this country. Such courses vary from several voluntary sessions to an entire semester of required work. Those of you who are not close to the school systems may not be aware that there is such a large group of health educators who, both in the school and in government agencies, have been taking over much of the work that has been historically that of physicians. Physicians have given it up under the plea of not having enough time. But it brings up a number of issues about who is responsible for certain aspects of education. I think we would all agree that all courses of this kind should be under the supervision of physicians and under optimal circumstances should be conducted by physicians. I can think of no more valuable, stimulating, and educational experience than to hear such questions as the ones I mentioned earlier in this paper and to attempt to deal with them. In organizing such courses, the issues of tact, direction, and planning are paramount. Parents must know about them; teachers must know about them. There must be a great deal of discussion of what is going to be done to prevent undercutting and bickering. In organizing such courses, experience suggests that boys and girls should be separated, though there have been a number of effective discussions of dating behavior conducted with boys and girls together.

In conducting such courses, a physician should be serious but not unctuous in his handling of material. There is very little place for talking with the voice of doom. The organization of the course should be definite and it should be filled with content and explicit words. We are not afraid of using them when we describe certain functions to teen-agers.

Because it is relevant to both the general discussion and specific involvements in the physician's office, I am going to outline one way to organize material on sexuality that is basic for a teen-ager to know. I will not spend any substantial time in discussing the larger meaning of sexuality in life, its relationship to tradition, morality, or religion, though I consider these aspects to be basic to sexual knowledge. Rather, I would anticipate that the very presentation and character of the physician giving such information would communicate his mature opinions on these crucial subjects.

Before a youngster is well into his teens, he should know about the anatomy and physiology of reproduction, the physical and emotional changes of puberty, and the variations in all of these.

The great question that a teen-ager has is, "Am I normal?" Young people need so much to be reassured that sexual feelings are normal and that great variations in the strength of feelings and in physical development of sexual characteristics are eminently normal. I could dilate on this theme but rather I will save a good deal of time for discussion and questions.

In addition to the physical and physiological material, teen-agers should be given a concept of acceptable dating behavior and of the restraints that are possible and healthy in dating behavior —manners, etiquette, the things that make a boy-girl friendship happy and what can spoil it should be included. The meaning of popularity and often the price of popularity should be stressed. There should be a discussion of the motivations that underlie various kinds of sex behavior, healthy and unhealthy, and the strength that comes from making up one's own mind rather than merely accepting the views of the majority. This naturally reaches back to parental concepts, but many children cannot depend upon their parents for much help in this area. We have to appeal to them directly. Instead of bypassing the issues of promiscuity, (and after Dr. Dougherty's presentation how can you possibly bypass those issues?) permissiveness, total abstinence, the various customs, one should have an opportunity to discuss views about them and the results of various kinds of behavior. The great differences between infatuation and love, between dating, going steady, and marriage should be enlarged upon. The importance of evaluating differences, particularly when going steady and marriage are involved, differences in religion, education, age, interests, socio-economic background, ethnic background, should be stressed for youngsters. These points can be illustrated through cases and a discussion of the very youngsters involved or from literary examples.

I will not attempt to discuss the issues involved in leading a group as they demand a great deal of attention. However, they are integral to what one does with a group of teen-agers. There are many publications which describe the techniques and strategy of developing group processes and of achieving an optimum openness without merely diffusing a group session.

The physician should be sure that youngsters know of the healthy importance and pleasure of sexuality as well as its dangers. Only at this time should the question of values be brought in. The physician should not be a preacher, but he also should not be an automaton who teaches as if sexuality were not a value charged function.

For example, he must point out that the girl always has final responsibility in how far she will go with a young boy. Girls frequently find themselves infatuated with boys who remind them of their fathers. They feel able to trust their fathers and therefore put great trust in a boyfriend. The boyfriend does not see himself in such a role at all, and, in fact, is often surprised and made anxious by a girl who leaves all the decisions to him. Particularly at this time in our country, it is important that a physician give teen-agers all the information that is available about sexuality, but, in addition, he should give his opinion that controls are absolutely necessary for many teen-agers, not only on religious grounds, but on the grounds of character development. That is, a boy caught up in sexual issues and uncertain about them has very little energy left to put into studies or other aspects of his life.

Frustration and impulse control are corner stones of further character development. The person who is able to strike a good balance between gratification and the necessary and healthy frustrations of life is the one who will deal with sexuality most successfully, as he is the one who will deal with eating, sleeping, working, or studying most successfully.

For the adolescent patient in the physician's office, it is obviously not possible to define so detailed a course. In fact, few adolescents come to physicians for such a course. However, it should be considered the physician's responsibility to explore the area of sexuality, though with the permission of the youngster's parents, as a regular aspect of his preventive medicine or well-child activity.

In the office, patients seldom volunteer sexual information or fears. The physician must ask about such issues. The significant negatives in regard to sexuality need to be emphasized, though we sometimes consider ourselves too sophisticated to do this. It is striking to read a study by Greenbank[1] in which he found that, of the 1959 graduates of all the medical schools in Philadelphia, "half of the students have a feeling that mental illness is frequently caused by masturbation. Even one faculty member in five still believes in this old, and now discredited, idea." There are also significant positives. It is no sin to counsel a patient, when it is appropriate, that kissing and happy romantic involvements should be happy aspects of growing up, both for boys and girls. The physician can emphasize that kissing and embracing can occur, but that touching the genital areas of boy or girl complicates and usually troubles relationships. This can be brought out in rational terms without invoking sin or dirtiness. Our experience with young teen-agers suggest that such a rule helps organize their behavior and prevents them from getting into exceedingly difficult positions of attempting to keep from going "all the way" while having allowed a great deal of body manipulation.

Once the youngster has begun to talk with the physician, the issue of confidentiality should be stressed. Much useful information can be learned or given through the use of leading questions. Instead of asking "Do you masturbate?"; the physician can say, "I guess masturbation has been a problem for you as it is for most boys." Even the silent patient can be given a general discussion of sexuality. In fact, most youngsters are all ears, even when they have said, "I don't know anything at all about those things." In this extraordinarily enlightened or at least sexually bombarded time, there are few children, boys or girls, who have not heard about masturbation or intercourse.

Naturally, the physician must look into his own heart and mind, to see what his views and prejudices are. He must also keep in mind that the patients he is counseling may well be the age of his own son or daughter. There is a great difference between the stance of a father of a fifteen-year-old girl going out on her first date and that of the physician talking with a seventeen-year-old girl who has come to him for the fitting of a diaphragm or information about the use of contraceptive pills. No father wants his daughter kissed by any boy, if you come down to that. It is a healthy response and the source of one of the great expected crises in everyone's life. Reflect on your views about teen-age girls. How many of you hope that your daughters will quickly get through the dating period and be "safely" married?

A final word about the general situation in this country in regard to sexuality. We are in ferment. The future orientation, the sense of stability, security, ambition, of accepted norms are all being attacked and in some case totally overthrown. We must recognize that the use of contraceptive pills is already a reality in many high school girls and may go much further. I do not wish to suggest any answers to these questions but believe that it is so much better to deal with issues, and in a knowledgeable way, than to hide from them. Many physicians are talking about sexuality as it existed when they were teen-agers. That is a long, long time ago for a fifteen-year-old of today. One of the best ways to be current in regard to the views and realities of sexuality with teen-agers today is to talk with them, interact with them, become involved in sex education courses in high schools. Only then, when a physician is well informed, can he exert a healthy and directing influence on the values and mores of the youngsters with whom he works.

These issues are significant ones for all our national organizations. The American Medical Association, the American Academy of Pediatrics, and many family service organizations have printed pamphlets and gotten materials together for the use of physicians. Such materials, however, should never be used as a short cut but rather as supplementary reading after actual discussion has occurred. In February of this year, a new organization, the Sex Information and Education Counsel of the United States, was started. Its roster of directors includes leaders of many religious groups and organizations concerned about sexuality. We can hope that, through SIECUS and other enlightened groups, sexuality will be considered in schools, homes, and physicians' offices in a more rational and effective way than it has been in the past.

REFERENCES

1. Greenbank, R. K.: Are medical students learning psychiatry? Pennsylvania M. J., *64:* 395, 1961.
2. Guest, H. H.: A report on sex education. Winnipeg School Division No. 1, Winnipeg, Canada, 1964.
3. Lief, H. I.: What medical schools teach about sex. Bull. Tulane Univ. Med. Faculty, *22:* 161, 1963.
4. Sandler, B.: The student and sex education. Lancet, p. 832. April 20, 1957.

Index

ACTH: see Adrenocorticotropic hormone
Adenoma of the adrenal, 97
Adolescence, definition of
  administrative, 1
  biological, 2
  psychological, 5
Adrenal adenoma, 97
Adrenal hyperfunction, as cause of virilization and hirsutism, 94
Adrenal hyperplasia, congenital, clinical manifestations, 92
Adrenal steroids
  metabolites of, 23
  production of, 22
Adrenal suppression test, use in differentiating between adrenal and ovarian androgen, 83
Adrenal tumor
  and hirsutism, 96
  urinary steroid excretion associated with, 97
Adrenocorticotropic hormone, action in production of steroids, 22
Alkaline phosphatase activity, changes at age 9, 10
Amenorrhea-menorrhagia syndrome in hirsute woman, 86
Amenorrhea
  nonpsychogenic, 45–57
  primary
    causes of, 50
    definition of, 49
    systemic diseases associated with, 50
  secondary
    causes of, 48
    definition of, 48
    psychogenic, 48
Androgenic activity
  growth of axillary hair as indicator of, 37
  seminal fluid as indicator of, 37
Androgens
  difficulty in measurement of, 40
  end-organ sensitivity to, 86
  evaluation by urinary steroid excretion patterns, 79
  in production of hypothalamic differentiation, 27
  in production of Wolffian differentiation, 27
  ovarian secretion, effect of human pituitary FSH on, 85
  role in hirsutism, 78
Androstenedione, in production of estrogens, 23
Anovulatory cycles, incidence of, 15
Arrhenoblastoma, 99
  description of, 73
Assays: see also specific assays
  criteria for evaluation, 34
  for identification of sex hormones, 33–44
Atrophic vaginal smear, significance of, 37
Axillary hair, growth as indicator of androgenic activity, 37

Barr body, in sex ambiguity, 60
Basal body temperature, relation to menstrual cycle, 16
Bio-assay
  and degree of correlation between human and nonhuman data, 36
  of progestational compounds, 38
Blood, as an indicator of steroid production, 25
BURNETT, A. M. Vaginitis, 104–108

Candida albicans, diagnosis of, 107
Chemical assays of steroid hormones, 38
Childbirth: see Pregnancy
Cholesterol, synthesis of sex steroids from, 22
Chorionic gonadotropin: see Human chorionic gonadotropin
Clitorectomy, as treatment for female pseudohermaphrodite, 62

Coitus, history of, associated with vaginal discharge, 106
Congenital defects, management of, 58–68
Cortisol, effects on androgenicity, 31
Cortisone therapy, for pseudohermaphrodites, 94, 95
Cyclic withdrawal bleeding, in treatment of metropathia hemorrhagica, 56
Cystadenofibroma, serous, description of, 72
Cystic tumor, 99
Cysts
  corpus luteum, 72
  parovarian, 72
  simple, 72
Cytology: *see* Urinary cytology

Dehydroepiandrosterone, complications in study of, 41
Denver classification, for sex determination, 60
11-Deoxy-17-ketosteroids, urinary, in normal and hirsute women, 82
Dougherty, W. J. Public health aspects of venereal disease, 109–129
Dysfunctional bleeding: *see* Metropathia hemorrhagica
Dysgerminoma, description of, 73

Education: *see* Sex education
Endocrinology, reproductive, 9–20
Endometrioma, description of, 72
End-organ sensitivity to androgens, 86
Epidemiologist, public health, role of in controlling syphilis, 121, 123
Estradiol
  excretion levels, 11
  uterine concentration, 24
Estriol, excretion levels, 11
Estrogen: *see also* specific estrogens
  absence of, associated with osteoporosis, 65
  activity in children, 10
  measurement of, 43
  output and karyopyknotic index of vaginal smear, 37
  urinary excretion of, 13, 14
Estrogen, urinary, variation of amounts excreted, 11
Estrone, excretion levels, 11

Fecundity, relation to age, 16, 18
Fibroma, description of, 72
Follicle-stimulating hormone
  detection of gonadotropic activity by means of, 10
  determination by immuno-assays, 36
  determination by Steelman-Pohley assay, 35
FSH: *see* Follicle-stimulating hormone

Gas chromatography, in measurement of 17-ketosteroids, 43
Girard reaction, use of in 17-ketosteroid determination, 42
Goldzieher, J. W. The identification of sex hormones by chemical and biological assays, 33–44
Gonad, dysgenetic, 91, 92
Gonadotropin
  activity in children, 10
  urinary excretion of, 11
Gonorrhea
  historical review of, 110
  reported U.S. cases: 1920–1965, 110
  reported U.S. cases: 1957–1964, 112
  unreported cases, 115
Graafian follicles, in girls under age 9, 10
Greenblatt, R. B.: *see* Mahesh, 77–103
Gynecological age, significance of, 46

Heald, F. P.
  Introduction, 1–4
  Ovarian tumors during adolescence, 69–76
Hermaphrodite
  example of, 61
  history of, 58
Hirsutism, 77–103
  and adrenal tumor, 96
  and androgen secretion, 79
  and plasma testosterone levels, 86
  as result of adrenal hyperfunction, 94
  endocrine factors, 78–100
  genetic factors, 77–78
  psychological factors, 30
  reaction to hormone treatment, 29
Homosexuality, and syphilis, 114, 115
Hormones: *see also* Endocrinology and the specific hormones
  biochemistry of, 21–32
  changes associated with menarche, 9
  differences in response to, 29

INDEX

secretion rates, isotope dilution method in measurement of, 44
Human chorionic gonadotropin, to demonstrate gonadotropic activity in children, 10
6-Hydroxycortisol, as an inhibitor of steroids, 22
Hyperplasia: *see* Adrenal hyperplasia
Hypertrichosis
  and ovarian tumor, 98
  atavistic, 78
Hypothalamic differentiation, androgens in production of, 27
Hypothyroidism, associated with hirsutism, 78

Immuno-assays, for FSH and LH determinations, 36
Infant size, effect of maternal age, 17, 18
Isotope dilution method, in measurement of hormonal secretion rates, 44

Karyopyknotic index of vaginal smear, correlation with estrogen output, 37
17-Ketosteroids
  as reflectors of adrenal function, 23
  determination of and Girard reaction, 42
  measurement of, 41
    by gas chromatography, 43

LH: *see* Luteinizing hormone
LLOYD, C. W. The biochemistry of steroids and hormones, 21–32
Luteal insufficiency, and deficient LH secretion, 14
Luteinizing hormone
  deficiency, reproductive consequences of, 14, 19
  detection of gonadotropic activity by means of, 10
  determination by immuno-assays, 36
  determination by ovarian ascorbic acid depletion test, 35

MAHESH, V. B., and GREENBLATT, R. B. Hirsutism, 77–103
MARANS, A. E. The psychological impact of pregnancy on the adolescent girl, 130–147
Maternity clinic, and unwed mothers, 131

Menarche
  as a biological marker, 3
  delayed, diagnosis of, 49
  relation to physiological parameters, 3
Menstruation
  abnormalities
    and prognosis for adult abnormality, 52
    and prognosis for adult fertility, 54
    as nonspecific symptoms, 45
    diagnostic methods, 50, 51
  erratic, implications of, 2
  normal adolescent pattern, 46
  relation of cycle to basal body temperature, 16
  pattern variations within individuals, 55
Metabolites of adrenal steroids, 23
Metropathia hemorrhagica, 45–57
  causes of, 47
  characteristics of, 47
  diagnosis of, 47
  treatment of, 56
Mosaics, causes of, 61
MCARTHUR, J. W. The reproductive endocrinology of adolescence, 9–20

Neisseria gonorrhoeae, 108
Norethynodrel, effect on estrogenic activity, 24

Oligomenorrhea, definition of, 45
Oophorectomy, effect on uterus in rats, 28
Orchiectomy, as treatment for male pseudohermaphrodite, 62
Osteoporosis, associated with lack of estrogen, 65
Ovarian ascorbic acid depletion test, for LH determination, 35
Ovarian cystadenoma
  pseudomucinous, description of, 71
  serous, description of, 72
Ovarian failure, diagnosis of, 51
Ovarian tumor, 69–76: *see also* specific tumors
  and hypertrichosis, 98
  clinical symptoms of, 74
  comparison of, in adolescents, adults, and children, 74
  masculinizing, clinical symptoms of, 98
  types and distribution of, 71–74

INDEX

Ovulation inducing drugs, 57
11-Oxygenated-17-ketosteroids, urinary, in normal and hirsute women, 82

Polycystic ovary syndrome
  as a reversible process, 32
  importance of early diagnosis, 7
Population, adolescent in the United States, 2
Pregnancy
  and reaction to body changes, 143
  denial of reality of, 145
  fear of abandonment in, 143
  fears of childbirth, 135
  increasing frequency of in adolescence, 130
  parental reaction to, 131, 137
  prenatal overeating, 136
  problems in prenatal care, 139
  psychological impact of, 130–147
  social results of, 133
Pregnanediol excretion by women, 17
Pregnanetriol, urinary, elevation in congenital adrenal hyperplasia, 92
Premarital examination, counseling during, 7
Progestational compounds, bio-assay of, 38
Progesterone, measurement of, 44
Prostatic weight method in determination of LH excretion, 12
Pseudohermaphrodite
  female
    definition of, 61
    treatment by clitorectomy, 162
  male, 90–92
    treatment by orchiectomy, 62
  results of cortisone therapy, 94, 95
Public health
  aspects of venereal disease, 109–129
  epidemiologist, role in controlling syphilis, 121

Reproductive endocrinology: see Endocrinology

Seminal fluid, as indicator of androgenic activity, 37
Serological tests for syphilis, 113
Sex ambiguity
  and the Barr body, 60
  and the Denver classification, 60
  and the "squash" technique, 60
  importance of early decision of sex of rearing, 59
Sex education, 148–157
  and dating behavior, 154
  basic information for a teenager, 153
  in the physician's office, 155
  need for, 149
  physicians' preparation for, 151
  through parents, 152
  through schools, 152
Sex hormones, identification by chemical and biological assays, 33–44
Sex steroid
  synthesis from cholesterol, 22
  secretion changes in adolescence, 11
Sexual exposure, high rate in Washington, D. C., 105
Sexual maturation
  relation to reproductive performance in chimpanzees, 18
  role of steroids, 27
Southam, A. L. Metropathia hemorrhagica and nonpsychogenic amenorrhea, 45–57
"Squash" technique for sex determination, 60
Steelman-Pohley assay, for FSH determination, 35
Stein-Leventhal syndrome
  etiology of, 89
  symptoms of, 89
  treatment by wedge resection, 56
  LH deficiency in, 19
  protective function, 19
Steroids, 31: see also Adrenal steroids, Sex steroids, Urinary steroids
  biochemistry of, 21–32
  clearance, 21, 23
  production
    indicators of rate, 25
    regulation of, 31
  role in sexual maturation, 27
  secretion, 21
  transport, 21
Steroid hormones, chemical assays of, 38
Sturgis, S. H.
  Introduction, 5–8
  The management of congenital defects, 58–68

INDEX

Surgical reconstruction
  importance of adolescent cooperation, 68
  importance of performing at an early age, 67
Syphilis
  age distribution of, 119
  and cluster interview, 125, 126
  and homosexuality, 114
  and serological tests, 113
  congenital, 113
    cases in New Jersey: 1963, 114
  contact, definition of, 124
  control, and public health epidemiologist, 121
  dark field examination of lesions, 122
  epidemic of, in city, 119
  epidemiological investigation of, 122
  geographical distribution of, 118
  historical review of, 109
  in homosexual males, 115
  private physician reporting of, 127
  ratio male to female cases of, 115
  reported New Jersey cases of: 1940–1965, 111
  reported U. S. cases of: 1920–1965, 110
  reported U. S. cases of: 1957–1964, 112
  treatment of "negative" contacts, 125
  unreported cases, 115

Teenagers, and venereal disease, 117
Teratoma-dermoid tumors, description of, 71
Testicular feminization syndrome, in hirsutism, 90
Testis, contralateral, 91, 92
Testosterone
  correlation with urinary ketosteroids in hirsute women, 28
  difficulty in measurement of, 40
  in production of estrogens, 23
  levels in normal women, 28
  plasma levels of, in hirsutism, 86
Tetrahydrocorticoids, urinary, in normal and hirsute women, 82
Thecal luteoma, description of, 72
Trichomonas vaginalis
  diagnosis of, 106
  treatment of, 106
Trichomonas vaginitis, 105
Tumor: *see* Adrenal tumor, Cystic tumor, Ovarian tumor, Teratoma-dermoid tumor
Turner's syndrome
  diagnosis of, 64
  psychological effects of, 66
  sexual results of hormone treatment, 67
  treatment of, 65

Urinary cytology, diagnostic aid in ovarian dysgenesis, 65
Urinary steroid excretion
  pattern
    as aid in androgen evaluation, 79
    comparison of in normal and hirsute women, 80, 84
    in hirsute women, 88
    in hirsute women with adrenal and ovarian hyperfunction, 87
    values associated with adrenal tumor, 97
Urine, as an indicator of steroid production, 25

Virilization, as result of adrenal hyperfunction, 94
Vaginal discharge
  degrees, of, 105
  results of cultures of, 106
Vaginal infections, 106–108
Vaginal smear: *see* Atrophic vaginal smear
Vaginitis, 104–108
Vaginitis, nonspecific, treatment of, 107
Venereal disease: *see also* Syphilis and Gonorrhea
  and teenagers, 117
  education, necessity of, 119
  public health aspects of, 109–129
  teenage, geographical distribution of, 120

Wedge resection, as treatment for Stein-Leventhal syndrome, 56
WERKMAN, S. L. Sex education in adolescence, 148–157
Wolffian differentiation
  androgens in production of, 27
  produced by androgen of fetus, 27

Zimmerman reaction, in measurement of 17-ketosteroids, 42